THE ONE STEP
FUNNEL

For Dentists

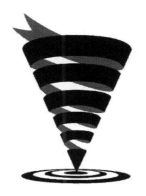

**How To Generate More High Value Dental Patients
Every Single Month by Attracting Your Ideal Patients,
Automating the Follow-Up Process, Scheduling More
Appointments and Closing More Sales!**

By Adam Braithwaite

One Step Funnel: How To Generate More High Value Dental Patients Every Single Month by Attracting Your Ideal Patients, Automating the Follow-Up Process, Scheduling More Appointments and Closing More Sales!

Copyright © 2019 Great White Media, LLC

Printed in the United States of America.

First Edition

Table of Contents

Dedication

I want to take a quick minute and thank all of those that have helped to make this book possible. From the countless trainers and coaches that in some way, either thru their training courses or live events have helped guide me on my journey to fully understanding and implementing all of the information in this book. Coaches and Trainers like Russell Brunson, Billy Gene, Sam Ovens, Matt Plapp, Robb Bailey, Amanda Becker and Chris Patterson are all incredibly talented at their craft and are the very best trainers and coaches in the world. Without your knowledge and persistent drive for your students to be successful, I would not have had the confidence to put that training into action.

I want to send a personal thank you to Billy Gene and the Billy Gene Is Marketing Team (specifically Rheya Green). Without your guidance, expertise and personal attention to this project, this book would not have gotten done. Thank you for holding me accountable and for bringing the clarity I needed to this project.

Finally, I want to thank my friends and family for their support and especially my two daughters, Sydney and Ava. Without your sacrifice of allowing me the time to work in my office for countless hours going through training courses, working with clients, listening to me talk about "Marketing, Sales and Funnel Strategies" and building my business, this would not have been possible. Through your support and encouragement, you continually drive me to be the best father, businessman and expert in my field that I can be. I love you both very much and always remember to not be afraid to give yourself everything you've ever wanted in life, but it takes great effort, determination, unwavering belief in yourself and personal sacrifice to achieve your dreams. I have no doubt you both will change the world and I want to thank you for allowing me to do my part.

Introduction

My name is Adam Braithwaite and I help Dentists reach their growth potential and dominate their local markets by implementing Our Proven Marketing System that generates More *Leads*, More Customers and brings in More Revenue. I have been in the marketing industry since 2004 and have been trained by world class trainers and coaches in marketing. Specifically local marketing techniques that leverages technology to achieve results. That way my clients can focus on what they do best; serve their customers.

I don't claim to be an "expert" because I continue to learn something new every day. All of the concepts in this book have come from my team and I working with clients and learning from other mentors in this industry. We took those concepts, put our own unique twist on it and applied our system to multiple clients all over the country. We put in the time and effort to build a Proven System we now call the "One Step Funnel".

What is the "One Step Funnel"?

We coined the phrase "One Step Funnel" because that's exactly how many steps it takes for the system to semi-automate the rest of the process. Have you ever heard a marketer talk about needing a "Sales Funnel"? Well, what they mean by that is a multi-step process of guiding a new lead to take a specific action. Maybe the process starts with a landing page that goes to a sales page that then goes to an upsell page and finally to a Thank You page. That's four steps to take and that's just too many steps for someone to have to go through to become a new patient of your Dental Practice.

What the One Step Funnel does is it Semi-Automates the entire process as soon as that potential new patient fills out and submits their contact information on a landing page. Once they do that, they would then get "Nurtured", which is a nice way of saying they get introduced to your Dental Practice through email, two-way text messages and ringless voicemails. We do that on the backend to get them to schedule an appointment. Once the appointment is scheduled, we then continue to nurture them with appointment reminders so that they show up to that appointment. It all starts with that potential new patient taking that One Step.

Who Is This Book For?

I wrote this book for those Dentists that want to take their practice to the next level. The Dentists that are tired of "lackluster" results from their marketing campaigns and want to finally figure out why their competitors are having a ton of success and they aren't. This book will uncover that for you. Be prepared to be humbled at first, but you will quickly regain momentum and see the whole picture of how the "One Step Funnel" is the key to your success.

What I Hope To Accomplish

The goal of this book is to not only explain the marketing systems that we use with our clients every day, but also what you can do to ensure your success. I want to explain what systems and processes you need to have in place to be successful at generating quality leads for your dental practice and how to properly nurture those leads to scheduling an appointment and to show up to that appointment.

Marketing Terms Used Throughout This Book

I know that some of the marketing terminology used in this book may be new to you. When you come across a bold and italicized word, that means that specific term is referenced in the "Marketing Terminology" section in the back of the book. Feel free to go there when you come across a word you don't recognize.

What's Next?

In the next chapter let's talk about the elephant in the room: Marketing Agency "Done For You" (DFY) vs "Do It With You" (DWY) or In-House and what one may be the best option for your Dental Practice.

www.OneStepFunnel.com

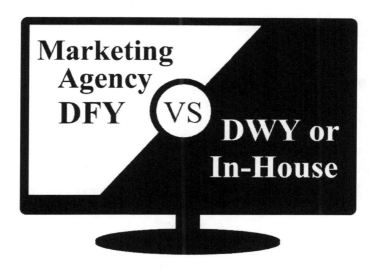

Marketing Agency DFY
vs DWY or In-House

> *"In order to succeed, we must first believe that we can."*
> *- Nikos Kazantzakis*

Many business owners are torn as to whether they should manage their lead generation in-house with an internal team or partner with a Marketing Agency. What's right for one Dental Practice might not be right for yours. How can you make the right decision? In this Chapter we will go through each one and why most Dental Practice's may be better off using a Hybrid Model instead.

Before we move on, I want to be clear that when you see the word "lead", "potential patient" or "potential customer", they are all the same thing. It's someone who gave us their contact information because they are interested in your Dental Practice and our goal is to get them to schedule an appointment with you. Ok, let's move on.

Marketing Agency DFY (Done For You)

A good Marketing Agency will handle everything from managing Facebook Ads to the ***Landing page***. From nurturing that lead all the way to scheduling an appointment. Literally, the only thing you should have to do is sell your services and let them know if the lead didn't show up. Everything else should be handled by the Marketing Agency. The only caveat to that may be the images of your practice and videos needed for the Ad Campaigns. Most Marketing Agencies require those to be provided by the client.

DWY (Do It With You)

With a DWY Program, basically it's everything that a Marketing Agency would do for you, but now you or your staff are doing it with the support of the Marketing Agency. This does require you or someone from your staff to be much more involved in the daily operation of Lead Generation and the Follow-Up Process.

You or your staff would be responding to leads and getting them to schedule an appointment. You would be building the Ad Copy, creating the images, running and managing the Facebook Ads and Reactivation Campaigns. Doing all of this with the support and oversight of the Marketing Agency. I know some of those terms may be new to you, don't worry, I will explain them in another chapter. The important part to know is that with DWY, you or your staff are doing everything with the support of a Marketing Agency.

In-House or DIY (Do It Yourself)

The issue with doing this In-House or DIY (Do It Yourself) is that you don't have the experience and support that the Marketing Agencies DFY or DWY Programs offer. You or your staff may not be trained in how it all works, and we see that most Dental Practice's that try it themselves end up doing more damage to their brand and lose a lot of money, then if they had a Marketing Agency to help them every step of the way.

The One Step Funnel Model

The One Step Funnel Program is a Hybrid of both DFY & DWY Programs.

The program starts out as a DFY Program (Done For You) with our team building out the Landing Pages, the *Email* Campaigns, Text Message Campaigns, we Setup the Google Sheet, Setup the Call Notifications and the Voicemail Drops. This usually takes up to 2-3 weeks depending on how quickly we get the digital assets and approvals back from our clients.

After the system is completely set-up, we transition into a DWY Program (Done With You) and schedule a one-on-one training session to show our clients how to edit and manage the system themselves and answer any questions they may have. We also give them access to the Training Portal that teaches our clients how to use the platform, how to add more follow up campaigns and effectively run and manage Facebook Ads. Once they start getting leads, we show them how to schedule the appointments on the Platform and nurture those leads all the way through to showing up to that appointment. At this point our role is more of a consultant and to offer ongoing support and staff training.

We do offer exclusivity and only work with one Dentist per 5-10-mile radius of their location. We do this because with our training we will help them DOMINATE that space and everyone in that area will know our client's Dental Practice, what they do and why they should go to them over anyone else in the area.

What Makes Us Different

What really stands out for us and what makes us very different from most Marketing Agencies, is that our system books the appointments for you. Most agencies simply deliver leads and hope they make an appointment, our system allows your staff to have two-way conversations with your potential patients and schedule the appointments for you. It really doesn't get any easier than that.

You can get more information about the One Step Funnel Program and see how it all works at: www.OneStepFunnel.com

Have You Ever Said This?

"I have a Marketing Agency that gives me leads, but those leads aren't any good."

First of all, if you have a Marketing Agency that's giving you leads, but you think those leads aren't any good, then why are you still paying that Marketing Agency in the first place?

Also, how are you following up with those leads? If you call the leads, how many times did you call them? Have you reached out via two-way texting? Have you sent any voicemail drops? If any of those are "NO", then it's probably not the leads, the issue is in the follow up. You have to fix the follow up system. The issue is that most "Marketing Agencies" don't have a Proven System that generates quality leads and nurtures them all the way through to coming into the appointment like we do.

What's Next?

In the next chapter we are going to talk about Why It's Important To Pay To Play. Businesses want consistency, and Paid Traffic can provide that consistent flow of new customers that you want, when done correctly.

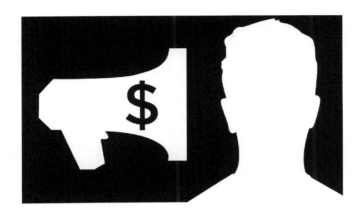

Why It's Important To "Pay To Play"

Before I get into this Chapter, I want to briefly explain how our Program works to generate leads. We have two ways we generate leads for our Dental clients.

The first way we generate leads is through running a "Reactivation Campaign". This is covered in detail in its own Chapter, but basically its where we take your current database or past customers and re-engage them to come back into your business. Your database is everyone that has ever come into your business for any of your services. Depending on the size of your database, this could account for up to 50% of your leads that you want every month. Obviously, the *offer* may be different than the Dental Implants example used in a later chapter, but we bring in patients for a variety of different services.

The second way we generate leads is through running Facebook Ads. The reason I wanted to bring that up now is so that you know that we supplement the Reactivation Campaigns with Facebook Ads to generate the amount of leads that you want each month.

Why "Pay To Play"

Pay-Per-Click Advertising or commonly referred to as PPC. Is probably the single most reliable traffic source that is present on the Internet today. The idea of PPC is actually pretty straightforward. As an Advertiser, you pay each time someone clicks on your Ad (Pay Per Click).

For Facebook, their PPC Ads are shown as "Sponsored" listings that show up in your newsfeed and other places you select, including Instagram. They show up in those places because the advertiser picked certain interests that the platform recognizes you have in common.

For example, if I liked "Nike" and an advertiser wants to show their Ad to men, ages 30-40 that like "Nike", then that Ad may be seen in my newsfeed because I fit all of the chosen criteria.

Benefits of PPC Marketing for Your Dental Practice:

1. Guaranteed Targeted Traffic.

2. Very Flexible Marketing Campaign (CPM or CPC bid). CPM stands for "Cost Per Thousand Impression" and CPC stands for "Cost Per Click".

3. Highest Value for Money (CPC can cost less than $1).

4. Access to Geo-Targeted Traffic.

5. Robust Advertising Technology.

6. Can be Started, Stopped and Adjusted Quickly.

It is so simple and fast to setup a PPC campaign on Facebook. This is the main reason why PPC marketing is also the most effective way to get traffic to any landing page. After an hour or so of putting up your Facebook Ad, you can expect people clicking on your Ad and going to your landing page.

PPC Provides Targeted Traffic

With Facebook Ads, you are provided an opportunity to pinpoint those individuals who have similar interests and show your Ads just to those people.

PPC Allows You To Change Your Ads Easily

With Facebook Ads you can change, edit, test and fine tune (optimize) your Ads to ensure that they will deliver the best results for you. If you think your existing Ad is not catching the attention of your target audience, then you can quickly change it until you get the right Ad Targeting, Ad Copy and Landing Page combinations. In the end, what PPC allows you to have is control over your Ads, the message you intend to deliver and the people you want to reach.

PPC Allows You To Test Your Campaigns Easily

With Facebook Ads, you can start a campaign, run an Ad Campaign for a few days and afterwards check the data to see if the campaign is really successful or not. If it wasn't, then you can quickly adjust it. You can easily run a split test (*A/B Testing*) and compare the campaigns to each other to see what is performing the best and stop the ones that aren't performing very well.

PPC Allows You To Reach More People

On Facebook, you will get a bunch of people seeing your Ad, we call that "Reach". The good thing is your Ad can be seen by thousands of people, but you only pay when someone clicks on the Ad. This is great for brand recognition too, because people are seeing your Ad even if they don't click on it.

PPC Allows You To Track Results

With Facebook Ads you can track your campaigns effortlessly and accurately on the platform. This allows you to tell whether a particular Ad campaign is efficient. It will tell you where your money was spent, even down to the last penny. This means you can determine **ROI (Return on Investment)** much faster with a PPC campaign. Facebook offers conversion tracking tools that you can use to track whether or not a campaign is making you money.

PPC Allows You To Have Geo-Targeted Ads

If you have a Dental Practice in Colorado Springs, for example, and you know that your clients live within the city limits, then it is useless to show your Ads to people outside of Colorado Springs. With Facebook Ads, you don't only get to choose where your Ads will be visible, what distance from an area you want to target, but you also get to choose when it will be displayed.

On Facebook and Instagram, you have the ability to target people a few different ways: "Everyone in this location", "People who live in this location", "People recently in this location" and "People traveling in this location". You can also place a pin on a map for your location and target people within a certain range from your location. As of right now it goes up to a 50 miles radius of the location you choose. Most Dental practices will stay within a 3-5 mile radius from their location with their targeting.

PPC Allows You To Schedule Your Ads

Most Dental offices have set weekly operating hours. With Facebook Ads, you are able to show your Ads during the working hours of your operation and disable it on the hours your practice is closed.

The One Step Funnel Approach To Facebook Ads

We run A LOT of Facebook Ads, but the benefit to our clients is that we use a Proprietary System to target their ideal patients. By doing that, this gives our clients a few key advantages over everyone else in their area. Since they are using our own Targeting Rules, we can market to these people as opposed to just a broad range of people in that area. We can Market to these people before anyone else can too. Which means we get to set the buying criteria and tell them why they should buy from us. We also get to be in front of these people more often because our clients Advertising Dollars are being used more effectively.

What's Coming Up next

I've had a ton of conversations with clients that want to hit a very high value goal each month on a shoestring budget. You can't expect to live in a Mansion but pay for a Motel or drive a Ferrari but pay for a smart car. It just doesn't work like that, so let's look at what you should expect to pay to reach your marketing goals. In the next chapter we are going to talk about Your Marketing Budget.

www.OneStepFunnel.com

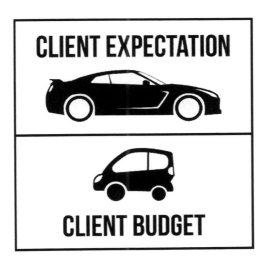

Your Marketing Budget

I've been to several Marketing Conferences, been in a bunch of Facebook groups with other marketers, listened to hundreds of marketing podcasts, watched countless hours of videos from a ton of different marketers and have had thousands of conversations over the years. You know what I have never heard any one of them talk about? They never talk about "Saving Marketing Dollars." In fact, besides spending money on coaches and further training to increase our knowledge, we spend more on "Marketing and Ad Spend" than anything else.

If you do an online search for a good marketing budget, you get a ton of different answers. You hear people make recommendations like 5% of Revenue, 10% of Revenue, 25% of Profit, etc. There are a lot of different answers. The fact is, there's no barometer to use to gauge what you should spend, but it needs to be as much as you can afford to spend to reach your goals.

We recommend to all of our clients that they spend as much as they can afford to spend on marketing. Generally, we don't work with less than $2,000 per month Ad Spend to start with. We like to start there and adjust either up or down depending on how many leads they get and how many leads the Dentist wants each month. One thing though, once you start Advertising, don't stop. If you don't need as many leads that month, simply lower your Ad Spend but keep the Ads turned on so the platform's algorithm keeps working to get you better leads.

Spend As Much Money As You Can On Marketing!

It's so affordable to get attention for your Dental Practice, you should be taking full advantage of this! Eventually, your patients will begin generating more and more business for you with warm referrals, but you always want to keep those cold leads coming in. Don't be cheap when it comes to spending money on your marketing. It's an investment and you will get out of it what you put into it.

Set Realistic Expectations With Your Budget

I hear it a lot at first with new clients, "I want XX number of "NP's" or New Patients each month, but can only afford to spend X." The issue with that way of thinking is that its completely backwards. The smart way of looking at it is to work the math backwards from how many new patients you want to take on each month and do the math to figure out the numbers. Below is an example of how we would do the math for our Dental clients.

The Assumptions

With our program we typically see that 70% of traffic will schedule an appointment. Through our Follow-Up Processes, we get on average about

70% of those appointments to show up to that appointment. Once a patient is in the seat, usually at least 60-70% will purchase the service. In this example though, let's be conservative and use a 50% close ratio.

Let's do an example of a Dental Campaign where the Dentist wants 20 New Dental Implant Patients per month.

The Math Worked Backwards

New Patients / Close Ratio = Appointments Needed To Show Up

We know that from our assumptions earlier, that we wanted 20 new Dental Implant patients. We also know that the Dentist should close at least 50% of those appointments. That means that 5 out of 10 appointments that show up would purchase Dental Implants.

20 / 50% = 40 Appointments Needed to Show Up

Appointments Needed To Show Up / Show Up Rate = Appointments Needed Per Month

Now that we know we need 40 overall appointments to show up, we have to figure out how many appointments we need to schedule each month. We know that a certain percentage of those will not show up to the appointment. From our assumptions, we said that 70% of the scheduled appointments will show up.

40 / 70% = 57 Appointments Needed Per Month

Appointments Needed Per Month / Schedule Rate = Leads Needed Per Month

Now that we know we need 57 total appointments scheduled per month, we have to figure out how many leads we will need to get that many appointments scheduled each month. We know that a certain percentage of those leads will not schedule an appointment. Just because someone fills out their contact information, doesn't mean they will book an appointment. Maybe it's not the right time or maybe they just wanted more information, either way some of them will not schedule an appointment. From our assumptions, we said that 70% of the leads will schedule an appointment.

57 / 70% = 82 Leads Needed Per Month

The End Result

In the end, you would need 82 new leads each month to get 40 appointments to show up. If you closed just 50% of them, which is way low, then you would get 20 new Dental Implant patients.

Next we have to figure out how much revenue those 20 NP's (New Patients) will bring in and deduct that from you marketing costs. If you normally charge $3,000 for a Dental Implant and had an Amazing offer of "$1,000 Off" like we would recommend, then the Net Revenue would be $2,000 per Dental Implant. Those 20 NP's (New Patients) would generate $40,000 in Revenue each month.

20 New Patients X $2,000 Per Dental Implant = $40,000 in Revenue

Let's just say that you spent a total of $8,000 on Marketing Agency/ Platforms + Ad Spend combined, you would still be ahead with a Net Revenue of $32,000 each month. That's a 400% Return on your Investment! I know, some readers may think that spending $8,000 in a month is a lot, but you can't go anywhere else and get that kind of return on your investment!

Let's put the ROI (Return on Investment) in perspective a little, shall we? Warren Buffett, the third richest man in the world at the time of this writing, has made his Billions by investing in the stock market. His average ROI during the last 50 years is 21%! How does that 400% return on your investment look now?

I know you still have to account for your overhead and other business expenses out of that $32,000, but in fairness, that number doesn't even include any of the upsells. Services like, hygiene appointments, teeth whitening, crowns, fillings, braces, other cosmetic procedures, referrals, etc. that happens naturally through proper *lead nurturing*.

With our program, initially we show our clients how to focus on the High Value Services to bring in a lot of revenue each month. However, as they nurture those new patients over time, we also get them in for other services as well. Oh, and you won't spend anywhere near the $8,000 per month on Marketing Agency/Platforms + Ad Spend combined with our program!

Now that we know we need to spend money on Paid Advertising, let's talk about how we get someone to take an action on our Ads. I like to call this the "bait" we use to get them to click on our Ad.

www.OneStepFunnel.com

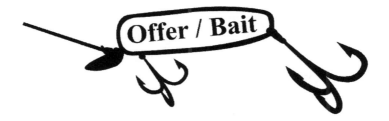

You Must Always Bait Your Hook

"Even when you are marketing to your entire audience or customer base, you are still simply speaking to a single human at any given time."
- Ann Handley

Let me tell you a quick story of a fishing trip I went on in July several years ago. A few of my friends and I had planned a five-day fishing trip to Lake Vermilion, Minnesota. We took several trips to Bass Pro Shops and Cabela's to get more fishing gear. We went all out and bought the big spinners, new rods and reels and some oddball lures that "had to work", or so we thought. We spent hundreds of dollars each on fishing lures for that trip, even before we left our driveway.

We did our research on the lake and figured out we were going after Walleye, the Northern Pike and that all to elusive fish they call the Muskie. We read articles about the kind of bait people used, we watched a ton of videos on YouTube and we bought something similar. I mean we were from Nebraska and it can't be much different up in the northern part of Minnesota, right?

Let me pause the story for a second and clue you in on how this relates to marketing. You see when you are looking for your ideal patient, it's kind of like going fishing. The fish in my story would be your ideal patient. We chose the type of fish we were going after and that's like you deciding on the type of patient you want to market too. Maybe it's the single moms or the people with a higher income, either way you choose who to target in your marketing. The bait we bought to try to catch the specific fish we were targeting is like the "Offer" we use in marketing to get that person to click on our Ad. Hopefully they bite the bait, or in your case they Opt-In to your funnel to get that offer.

Ok now, back to my fishing story. Once we drove up to Lake Vermillion, we couldn't wait to get the boat into the water. One of my friends wanted to stop by a bait shop, so we stopped in to see if they could give us any tips of where the big fish are biting. When we went into the bait shop, the guy who was working there asked if we were here for the skiing tournament? We said no, we were here for a guy's fishing trip. He semi-politely laughed and said, "No one goes fishing here in July!" He said the only thing that works this time of year are minnows. If you want to catch Northern Pikes, use this spinner. You know what, he was right! All those nice expensive lures didn't catch a single fish. But the minnows, caught a ton of Rock Bass and that specific spinner did catch several Northern Pikes for each of us.

You see, the critical mistake we made was not using the right bait to catch the fish we wanted. Throwing out the wrong bait didn't catch us anything. As soon as we used the right bait, we started catching fish like crazy. Sometimes, you have to adapt and go with what is working at that moment in time.

Bringing this back into the marketing side, if you know who you are targeting and put the right offer in front of that person at the right time, most of the time they will take it. Occasionally, you can have the right offer, the right target market, but for whatever reason it's not the right time for that person to take you up on that offer. It's ok, not everyone will need your services all of the time. What is important is that you are constantly putting up new offers to get the right bait in front of that person.

I remember the first time I saw a Muskie on that fishing trip. It was hovering there by some seaweed and it was about a foot below the top of the water. At least that's what we thought, when we all were amazed at how big it was in the water. It was maybe 5 feet from the boat and looked like a four-foot log staring at us. The funny thing was, each of us had a different lure for that fish and we slowly pulled it right in front of that fish's mouth. We must have been just a few inches from its mouth and it didn't take the bait. No matter what bait we used it just wasn't interested. A few minutes of this and finally that huge fish swam away.

The point of that story is that you never know what offer or bait will work. If we use the same bait and expect it to work on everyone, you won't catch very much. The best thing to do is have a specific offer to each target audience you are marketing too. You can use the same offer for multiple different audiences, but just know that you always have to match the offer with the target audience for a marketing campaign to have a chance at it working.

In marketing, this applies to several different areas of the customer journey. We use one kind of bait or offer incentive to get them to click on our Ad. If it's not engaging or powerful enough, they won't click on it and we won't get the traffic we need.

Once they click on the Ad, we use that same bait or offer to give them what they wanted. It's amazing to me how many businesses do a "bait and switch" type of thing with their Ads. Don't ever do this! If someone clicks on an Ad for a "$1,000 Off of Dental Implants" from a Dentist for example, don't send them to a page about your business. That's not a good "Offer to Market Match". They clicked on the Ad for a "$1,000 Off of Dental Implants", not to learn that you went to a specific college and that you have an amazing staff. Send them to a page about how to claim their "$1,000 Off of Dental Implants" coupon.

Another time we use the "Offer to Market Match" is through our Automation Sequences. We will be going over those in a later chapter, but for now I want you to know that you must always have an "Offer to Market Match" to be successful in marketing.

Why You Need A Spectacular Offer To Stand Out

We like to focus on what brings in the most revenue for our clients. Typically, that means they want Dental Implant patients, Cosmetic patients or even braces.

Where most Dental Practices set themselves up to fail, is that they price their services the same as everyone else in their market. I know, this sounds counter-productive right? I mean, why would anyone have their prices set higher than everyone else. The answer is: To Stand Out!

Think about it for a minute, if everyone charges $2,500 for a Dental Implant, what are the offers that you and everyone else use? "$500 off Dental Implants", you see it everywhere all the time. How do you stand out in that situation? You don't. You can't, because you have no room in your pricing structure to make a better more enticing offer.

However, if you raise your price to $3,000 or $3,500 per Dental Implant and go to market with a "$1,000 Off Dental Implant" coupon, while everyone else is still offering that $500 Off coupon, who do you think is going to stand head and shoulders above everyone else? You are! It's important to think how you can stand out from everyone else in the market, but at the same time not give away all of your profits either. No one wants to work for free.

This is sometimes a sticking point for some Dental Practitioners, but your marketing will suffer greatly if you just blend in with every other Dental Office in your area. In fact, when we interview our clients to see if they would be a good fit for our program or not, we talk about this in detail. The fact is, if they aren't willing to change their prices to give us an

Amazing offer to work with, then it's usually not a good fit for either of us to work together.

Now that we know that our offer is extremely important and used in several places, let's look at a complete local marketing system we call the One Step Funnel Program in the next chapter.

www.OneStepFunnel.com

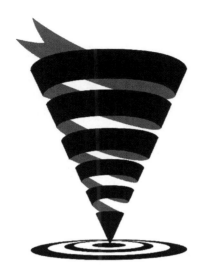

The One Step Funnel Program

"Do one thing every day that scares you." - Eleanor Roosevelt

---

A complete marketing system should encompass everything from finding the ideal patient to nurturing that potential patient to setting the appointment and finally getting them to show up for that appointment. Your process may have a few more steps or could even involve less, but the point is that a complete marketing system should cover everything.

The One Step Funnel Program starts with figuring out who your ideal patient is and how much you want to invest in your marketing budget. Notice I said "Invest", not "Spend". Marketing should be considered an investment, not just a simple business expense. The next step is to get "traffic" (website visitors or potential customers) through Facebook Ads. After that, the next step is the Automation Steps that we use to nurture that new lead. This stage in the process is one of the most powerful parts of the whole program and will play a key role in deciding if you will be successful in your marketing efforts or not. This will semi-automate how you follow up with that new lead on a variety of different platforms. We will incorporate Two-Way Text Messaging, Ringless Voicemails, Emails and Live Calls from the staff. Through these different channels, our goal is to get them to schedule an appointment and come into your practice for that appointment. Finally, assuming you made the sale, we will ask for an Online Review on either Facebook or Google. All of this is done, while continuously nurturing this new lead to become a raving fan of your dental practice.

The One Step Funnel

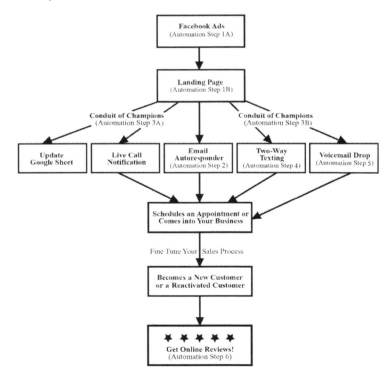

In the following chapters, this is what I will be explaining. I know it may look complicated, but it's important for you to understand how Our Program works so you can decide if this is something you want for your practice.

We Address People's Fear of Dentistry Throughout The Nurturing Process

It's estimated that seventy-five percent of adults in the United States experience some amount of fear with regards to visiting the dentist. By recognizing that and embracing this, we can build out the nurturing program to help alleviate some of those fears. It's important to build a rapport and trust with each new lead and we do that through providing valuable *content* and making them feel welcome at your dental practice.

How Do We Not Overdue The Automation?

We sometimes hear the question of "With that many follow-ups with each new lead, wouldn't they get tired of receiving them and get upset?" When does it become "too much"? The answer is, it depends. It depends if you have it setup correctly or not. You want certain delays in each different type of contact and you also want to have it be at certain times too. There definitely is a fine line that needs to be addressed and that's what we cover in detail in the Training portal for our clients. We have the experience and history that goes with managing this system so we can help set it up properly and it has a natural feel to it.

How to Use This Book to Be Successful

I wrote this book to explain what the One Step Funnel Program is and how it could be used for your business. You can get more information about the One Step Funnel Program at: www.OneStepFunnel.com

Because you are reading this book and have gotten this far, that shows that you are committed to your success. As a way to say Thank You, I wanted to give you something special to help you succeed even more and to show my commitment to your success. There is nothing more precious than time, so I would like to invite you to go to www.OneStepFunnel.com and Schedule a FREE Strategy Session with one of our Team Members.

On this call we will discuss your Overall Marketing Strategy and see how we can implement the One Step Funnel Program into your Dental Practice. Every business is different, and our goal is to deliver massive value to you during the call. It's important for you to know what's working right now and how you can implement those strategies into your business. If you are a good fit for the program, then we will figure out the best way for us to get started working together. We can't offer this to everyone and only accept a limited number of new clients each month, so be sure to schedule your call before we fill up.

I know from experience that by simply asking someone to go to a website and register for a FREE Strategy Session, that a certain percentage of people won't even do that. What that does, is it helps weed out those people that won't put in the effort to get the results they can achieve and are usually hard to work with. Please don't be one of those people that just read the book and doesn't take action. Conrad Hilton once said, "Success seems to be connected with action. Successful people keep moving. They make mistakes, but they don't quit." Simply reading this book and taking an action by Scheduling a FREE Strategy Session with one of our Team Members shows that you are committed to your success!!

What To Expect From The Rest Of The Book

Let's take a look at what each of the following chapters will cover:

Choosing Your Ideal Patient: Here we will look at what your ideal patient looks like and how to figure that out. We can use this information to target specific groups or similar people with your Ads that share common interests.

Automation Step 1A: Facebook Ads: Here we will look at why Facebook and Instagram Ads should be your main source of paid traffic to your business. We use Facebook Ads two different ways and we will cover that in this chapter.

Retargeting: Capture Those Leads That Were Interested: Here we will look at those leads that maybe clicked on our Ad but didn't fill out the *online form*. Maybe they looked at your website but haven't called to make an appointment or haven't taken a specific action yet. Those people can be targeted specifically with a Retargeting Campaign, meaning our Ads would just be shown to those people. This has tremendous power and if used correctly, will act as a safety net to capture those prospects that were interested at one time and try to re-engage them.

You Have Traffic, Now What?: In this Chapter, we go over where to send that Traffic to and how we follow up with those new leads. This is one of the biggest mistakes most DIY Marketers do that almost guarantees that they fail. The fortune is in the follow up! You would be amazed at how many times a new lead is never followed up with. Here we go over what you or your staff should be doing to make sure that every lead gets handled properly.

Automation Step 1B: The Opt-In Funnel: This is where we will send the vast majority of our Paid Traffic too. The Ad copy will match the Opt-In page and therefore give the potential new customer only one choice on this page, either do what we ask (submitting their contact information) or leave.

Automation Step 2: Email Autoresponder: This is one of the ways we will use to nurture that new lead and begin to build credibility with them. Think of this as a three-pronged approach to each new lead. We will use Email, Two-Way Text Messaging and Ringless Voicemails to automate the follow up process.

Automation Step 3: The Conduit of Champions: This is the glue that ties everything together. This part of the Automation process allows us to have multiple things going on in the background simultaneously. This all starts when someone fills out their contact information on your Opt-In page.

Automation Step 4: The Power of Texting: This is the second prong of our three-pronged approach to follow up. Texting is by far one of the most effective channels of communication with a new lead. Not everyone will answer a phone call from a phone number they don't recognize, however studies shown that almost everyone will read a text message from that same number.

Reactivation Campaigns: This is how we will "Reactivate" or re-engage with past customers to bring them back into your business. This is the tool that "Marketing Agencies" use when they say that they can get leads with "Zero Ad Spend".

Automation Step 5: Ringless Voicemail: This is the third prong of our three-pronged approach to follow up. We also will use this as a way to give a personal message to our contacts. Sometimes, hearing a voice and getting a message from a business is what makes the difference between you and your competition.

Non-Automated Tasks & Your Sales Process: In this Chapter we talk about what can't be automated and how to effectively manage these tasks. We also talk about your sales process and why you should have a defined process in place.

Automation Step 6: Get Online Reviews!: This is critically important and often overlooked by most "Marketing Agencies" and business owners. Online review sites and even Facebook and Google reviews are so important for your Ads, local searches and even your local maps listings.

Over time, this one thing could potentially be responsible for almost all of your new leads coming in. It's that important!

Putting It All Together: Here we explain how all of these pieces fit together in perfect harmony. It's like a well-oiled machine when setup correctly. This is the part when all of the other Chapters come together, and you will see the Big Picture.

The next chapter will start the One Step Funnel Program by Choosing Your Ideal Patient.

www.OneStepFunnel.com

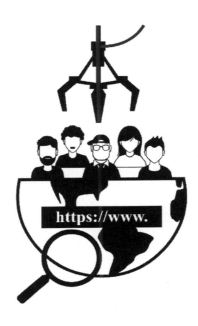

Choosing Your Ideal Patient

"The way to get started is to quit talking and begin doing." - Walt Disney

The first part of the One Step Funnel Program is to choose your ideal patient. We sometimes will refer to this as the "Crane", a thank you to Billy Gene Is Marketing for the reference. The reason we call it a "Crane" is because this is where you tell Facebook who you want to target. You hand select certain interests and characteristics to narrow down your ideal customer, the people you want to serve in your Dental Practice.

This is similar to the Claw Game at many toy shops or vending machine areas that have the claw that comes down to try to grab a small toy. The joystick that you move around is like you choosing your ideal customer by selecting characteristics that your ideal customers all would or should have in common.

The characteristics such as: Age group, male or female or both, interests, things they like, people they would follow, etc. All of this will help narrow down a group of people into an "audience".

Then when you hit that red button on the top of the joystick and it goes down to try to pick up that toy, that's when you see how effective your choices are. Marketing is very much like that. You get to decide who to target based on your best guess or a survey of your current patients. It's highly recommended that you have your patients fill out a survey asking them questions about how they heard about your business, what services they like or wished you offered, what was their experience like, interests they have, people they follow, TV shows they watch, music they listen too, etc. It may seem weird to ask all sorts of questions, but the more information you can get, the better and the more targeted your marketing campaigns can be.

Every Dental Practice is different in one way or another. However, most Dentists I meet with tell me their favorite demographic is the 30 something year old's that want the benefit your offer can bring them, earns a good income and lives within a few miles from their dental office. Something similar to that is pretty much the standard targeting for dentists.

Typical Traditional Online Marketing Methods

Ok, so I'm going to use another "Fishing Analogy" to explain the different platforms and what you can expect to receive by using those platforms. Afterwards, I'm going to explain what we do differently.

Radio & Television

When I think about Radio and Television Ads, I picture someone swimming in the water trying to catch fish with their bare hands. That is what Dental Practices did in the 90's with Radio and TV Ads. They may have gotten a few leads, but it's a lot of money and work for what little they got out of it.

Radio & TV

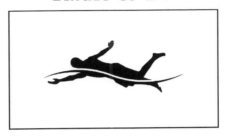

Search Engine Optimization (SEO) & Local Search

When I think about Search Engine Optimization (SEO) & Local Search, I picture my friends and I dragging a net and positioning our entire business on top of a search engine. When you do that, every other business that you are competing against will also come up in the search engines with you. Imagine being just one of the top five Dental Practice's that show up in the search results.

SEO & Local Search

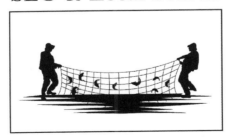

Google Ads

If we want to change things up a little bit, we will use Google Ads occasionally. Google Ads reminds me of getting in my little boat and using an expensive bait to cast out my offer. Your cost to acquire a new patient is a little higher, but you are targeting specific "buyer keywords".

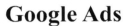
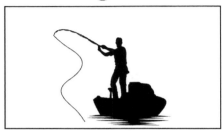

What We Do Differently

During the Marketing Phase of our program, one of the first things we do with our clients is we have them purchase a detailed list of names, email and phone numbers of people that have purchased specific services in their local area. We use "Purchase Behavior" technology to help fine tune the targeting for their Facebook Ad Campaigns. This would be like spearfishing in a swimming pool. We can get information on people that are in your community that can afford your services and that have shown some kind of indication they bought or are interested in your services. That is EXTREMELY Powerful!

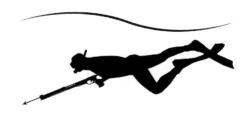

This little trick will drastically reduce your CPC (Cost Per Click) because it's what the Big Businesses use to show Ads to specific individuals in an area. Most Marketing Agencies don't use this technology or even know how to get it. We have access to this technology through our business connections we have developed, which gives us a Huge Advantage in the marketplace and our clients end up paying a lot less cost per click because of it.

OK, we have our target or ideal customer in our sights and have created multiple audiences to target with our "Crane". Now what? In the next chapter, I'm going to go over Automation Step 1A: Facebook Ads.

www.OneStepFunnel.com

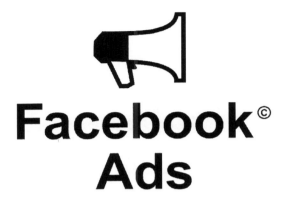

Facebook©
Ads

Automation Step 1A: Facebook Ads

"Our jobs as marketers are to understand how the customer wants to buy and help them do so." - Bryan Eisenberg

---

This is one of the two ways we generate leads. It's no secret that social media is dominating modern society. Most of us know this because you (like me) probably check your Facebook, Instagram, and Twitter feeds numerous times throughout the day. Well, guess what? Your customers do the exact same thing.

There is one social network that ALL marketers and business owners simply can't ignore, and that is Facebook. Don't believe me? Well, let's take a look at five reasons why you should below. Before we do that though, let me tell you that Facebook owns Instagram. So, when we are talking about Facebook, it also refers to Instagram since you have the option to run the Ad on Instagram from Facebook's platform. OK, so now that we know those two are on the same team, let's look at the five reasons why we use Facebook Ads as our preferred Paid Traffic Source to supplement our Reactivation Campaigns.

#1: Your Audience Is on Facebook

Facebook has a user base bigger than the population of China! With 2.27 billion active members worldwide, Facebook is presenting businesses with the greatest advertising opportunity since we could browse the internet. So yes, your audience is on there someplace, it's just a matter of locating them (which I'll go into in reason # 3).

#2: Facebook Ads Are Inexpensive

Truly, they are pretty affordable compared to other sources of traffic. The average cost per click is about $1.72. Please note that depending on how good the offer is, how good the targeting is, it may take several clicks to get a single lead.

#3: The Targeting Capabilities of Facebook Are Phenomenal

In addition to lots of different Ad types, the level of detail you can drill down to with Facebook targeting capabilities is unbelievable. Regardless if it be by behavior, interests, demographics, connections, age ranges, languages, or locations, you can dig pretty deep with these targeting capabilities and stack them on top of one another to ensure you're removing any questionable, out-of-market clickers.

*** *Please note that Facebook is constantly updating its Targeting Rules. What that means is that they will add new targeting options and also will remove them as well. So, it's very important to stay up to date with your Ads to make sure they are running correctly. <u>We are constantly updating the Training Portal with Facebook's updates and Targeting changes so our clients can stay current.</u>* ***

#4: Facebook Is Efficient at Pushing Leads Down the Funnel

Experiment with remarketing on Facebook through custom audiences. I talk more about this in detail in a later Chapter. This strategy works good for marketers because remarketing works by targeting an audience that has previously visited your site, and for that reason is more likely to be interested in your products or services to some degree.

#5: Facebook Makes It Possible For You to Find New Qualified Leads Easily

Once you've found an audience that converts well, you can duplicate them. The feature is called "lookalike audiences" where you can take a custom audience and Facebook will search for and reach NEW people who resemble that audience and as a result likely to become interested in your business.

The Two Ways We Use Facebook Ads

We use Facebook Ads two different ways. You can use Facebook Ads to send someone that clicks on your Ad to a Landing Page (Automation Step 1B), which is what we do most of the time. The second way we use Facebook Ads is a little more advanced because of how to set it up each time, but we use Facebook Lead Ads.

Facebook Lead Ads allow advertisers to collect information from prospects directly from mobile ads. Instead of sending traffic to a landing page where people manually fill out a form and press submit, they click on the ad, their information (name, email & phone number) is pre-populated, and they hit submit. All within the Facebook platform. By doing this, you can also tie in the other Automation Steps in our program using Facebooks Third-Party Integrations and our "Conduit of Champions" (Automation Step 3). The downside of Facebook Lead Ads is that you have to setup all the Automation Steps each time you create a Facebook Lead Ad.

I know that some people like to just use Facebook Lead Ads, but the downside is that sometimes you want to give someone more information about your offer after they clicked on your Ad. A Landing Page (Automation Step 1B) allows you to do this and that's why we use it most of the time for our clients. We do use both, but more often that not we use a Landing Page.

In the "Putting It All Together" chapter, I will show you both diagrams, that way you have a visual representation of how Facebook Ads fit into our program.

Have You Ever Said This?

"I tried Facebook Ads before and it doesn't work for me..."

I love this response because when I ask if they have a Facebook *Pixel* on their website, they don't know what I'm talking about. When I ask if they have ever run retargeting campaigns before, again, I get a blank stare. When they tell me, they send their paid traffic to their website, I smile and agree that the way they ran their Facebook Ads before wouldn't work for them.

This is usually where they either take it upon themselves to get educated about how to do it successfully or they hire an outside firm to handle it for them. I know it took several years before you became a Dentist and you were proficient enough at it to be considered an "expert". The same is true for your marketing efforts. You could spend a lot of time and money to try to get proficient at it yourself, but even then, what "works now" changes constantly. That's why we are constantly updating our Advertising Strategies inside the Training Portal for our clients.

Now that you know more about Facebook and Instagram Ads, in the next chapter we are going to talk about what happens when someone goes to our landing page or clicks on our Ad and doesn't become a new lead. One of my mentors, Billy Gene, calls this the "Safety Net" of our marketing campaigns.

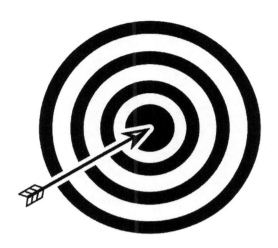

Retargeting: Capture Those Leads That Were Interested

Retargeting, also referred to as remarketing, is a form of online advertising that can help you put your business back in front of traffic after they leave your website. For most websites, only 2% of web traffic converts on the first visit. Retargeting is a tool created to help companies reach the 98% of users who don't convert immediately.

How Does Retargeting Work?

Retargeting is a *cookie-based technology* that uses basic *JavaScript* code to anonymously 'follow' your audience around the Internet.

Here's how it works, you install a small, unnoticeable piece of code on your website (this code is often referred to as a pixel). The code, or pixel, is unnoticeable to your site visitors and won't affect your site's functionality. Each time a new visitor goes to your site, the code drops an anonymous browser cookie. Later, when your cookied visitors browse the Internet, the cookie will let your retargeting provider know when to serve Ads, ensuring that your Ads are served to only people who have already visited your site.

Does Retargeting Work?

The answer is a definite YES!

Retargeting is so effective because it focuses your advertising dollars on people who are already aware of your Dental Practice and have recently shown interest. That's why the majority of marketers who use it see a higher ROI than from most other digital activities.

Various studies have shown that Retargeting Ad campaigns result in a steep rise in *conversion rates*. They can increase Ad responses by up to 400%!

Further, Retargeted Ads can not only influence visitors for a direct response, they can also improve brand awareness and recall.

Here are some more data points to support Retargeting effectiveness:

1. The average *click through rate* for Retargeted Ads is 10 times greater than the *click through rate* for regular Ads.

2. Website visitors who are served with Retargeted Ads are 70% more likely to make a conversion (Conversion means they take a specific action, like filling out a form, making a purchase).

3. Retargeting can lead to a 147% higher conversion rate, when used in combination with prospecting.

When Does Retargeting Work?

Retargeting is an effective branding and conversion optimization tool, but it works best if it's part of a larger digital strategy.

Below are a few ways you can use Retargeting:

Email Retargeting: Serving Ads to people who open (or interact with) your emails. You can segment the audience on the basis of different email types that you send: introductory emails, product-info emails, promotional email, etc.

Search Retargeting: Serving Ads to people who search for specific products on search engines.

Social Retargeting: Serving Ads to people who interact with your posts on social media (through likes, tweets, comments, and shares). You can segment the audience on the basis of different post types and the different actions users have taken on the posts.

How Our Clients Use Retargeting Ads

We start to run Retargeting Ads once we have enough data to build an "Audience" for Facebook's Algorithm. What this does is it allows our clients to split up the Ad Budget into a few different categories. They can use a portion for new traffic and another portion to bring that traffic that didn't convert back to their Opt-In Funnel.

In the next chapter, You Have Traffic, Now What, we are going to look at what happens when we use Facebook Ads to send someone to a Landing Page.

www.OneStepFunnel.com

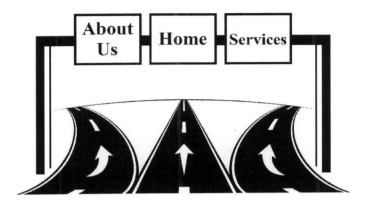

You Have Traffic, Now What?

"Some people dream of success, while other people get up every morning and make it happen." - Wayne Huizenga

Now that we know that we get part of your traffic from Facebook Ads, let's talk about what you should do with that traffic. In the following chapters we are going to talk about where to send the traffic to and what to do after it converts into a lead.

When you run paid advertising campaigns, you need to send that person to a specific web page or Opt-In Page, that gives them exactly what they clicked on. This is the "Offer to Market" match we talked about in a previous chapter.

Once that person fills out the contact form on your Opt-In page, also referred to as a "Landing Page", that will start the rest of the Automation Steps in the One Step Funnel Program.

We Will Never Send Paid Traffic To Your Website

You made your website to attract potential customers and leads online, so do you really need to have more web pages? It's appealing to set up your website and check the online lead box crossed off. Unfortunately, this is not the case. When it comes down to a landing page vs website, your website is your whole online first impression, while your landing page is just one component of that impression; it's your handshake, a nice greeting, or smile. You need both to make your online first impression really powerful.

Landing Page vs Website: The Basics

Website: Your website is a set of connected pages with detailed information about your business. Typically, Dental websites describe who they are, what services they offer and directions on how to get there. They can even contain other pages such your business blog, patient reviews or an image gallery. The main function of a website is to describe and explain your Dental Practice.

Landing Page: A landing page is created for one purpose, usually to explain an offer, maybe a discount coupon, or a free trial and encourage visitors to Opt-In to get it. Though it's linked to the website, it highlights important elements concentrated on conversion and does not have navigation buttons or other links. The primary purpose of a landing page is to capture leads. No other "distractions" go on a landing page or Opt-In page, it's incredibly narrow focused so the visitor takes that one specific action or leaves.

Our High Converting Landing Page Model

In our program we build a series of high converting Landing Pages for our clients. Each page is designed for a specific offer and geared to attract and capture new leads. We do that so we can build a list of highly targeted prospects and send them information based on what they want to know.

Each page has a click to call feature for mobile phones, a button to schedule an appointment and a button to instantly start a Two-Way Text Conversation with one of your staff members. It by far outperforms any Dental Website we have come across.

These landing pages are meant to capture new leads from traffic you control, such as paid traffic or social media posts, etc. We do this so that you can always send your paid traffic to a specific landing page that matches the offer in your Ad instead of your website.

Statistics from Our Own Testing

OK, let's stay away from theoretical situations and just talk facts. Our stats show that we convert 6X more traffic into leads when we send them to a well-structured landing page versus your standard website. Typically, a decent website will convert 4% of its traffic. A landing page typically converts 20-25%, but we've seen up to 45% in some cases.

Another great feature of landing pages is we can do split testing or also known as A/B testing. This means we can create your landing page, then duplicate the page and have a second version that we can change something on and send equal traffic to (50/50) and see which version works best. After that, we pick the winner, duplicate that one, and make another change. Then we just rinse and repeat until we reach the highest converting version of that page we can get and just keep paying to send traffic there!

This A/B testing method is also used when developing Ads to see which version of the similar Ads generate a large number of clicks at the lowest cost. Since we are A/B testing your Ads and A/B testing your landing pages, we are already leaving the majority of your competitors in the dust.

Have You Ever Said This?

"But I have a website, do I really need an Opt-In Funnel?"

Great question, and I know we just covered this, but I want to go through an analogy with you to really solidify the difference between a website and a landing page.

When a person lands on your homepage of your website it's kind of like a four-lane highway, and each page on the website is kind of like off ramps... Traffic (also referred to as website visitors) are going everywhere.

Some traffic visits the about us page, other traffic may visit a blog post, and some traffic may head to a services page to book an appointment.

Unfortunately, those streams of traffic are taking off-ramps from the main homepage ... Often times, if the visitor doesn't find what they are looking for, they leave and may never come back.

The biggest problem with website's is the visitor has a variety of choices with no obvious path to navigate.

So, how can an Opt-In Funnel solve this problem? I want to circle back to my analogy of roadways to explain an Opt-In Funnel.

Think about an Opt-In Funnel as a type of website that is kind of like a set of one-way streets.

All traffic is heading one direction towards the same goal of making a sale... With an Opt-In Funnel, there aren't links to other web pages or social media share buttons to distract the visitor.

The fact that there is only one thing for visitors to focus on is what makes the Opt-In Funnel different than a website ... Each page of an Opt-In Funnel has one objective, and the visitor either completes that objective or leaves.

Now, you might be thinking how does that benefit my business?

By removing distractions for the visitor, they can focus on what you are offering, which leads to higher sales conversions (something everyone wants, right?).

In the next chapter, we are going to look at Automation Step 1B: The Opt-In Funnel.

www.OneStepFunnel.com

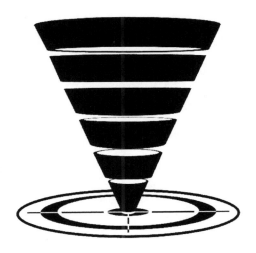

Automation Step 1B: The Opt-In Funnel

I'm super excited about this Chapter because this starts the Automation part of the One Step Funnel Program.

Ok, so let's assume that we are going to be generating traffic through Facebook Ads. To run our Ads effectively, we need somewhere to send that traffic to that has the perfect "Offer to Market" match we discussed earlier.

The place we want to send this highly targeted traffic to is an Opt-In Funnel, specifically the landing page. That way the person who lands on this page has just one task to complete, provide your name, email and phone number to get our special offer on the next page or leave. That's all we want to have on this page. Now, you will need to have a few additional pages setup as well to be in compliance with the Ad Networks, but these are pretty basic.

Let's clarify something, the term "Opt-In Funnel" refers to the entire system of web pages. The "Landing Page" is the first page in our "Opt-In Funnel". Similarly, the "Thank you Page" is the second page in our "Opt-In Funnel". We also would need some standard language and links at the bottom for compliance purposes like: Privacy Policy page and a Terms & Conditions page. Those are considered "Sub-pages" since they are part of the same domain but aren't a part of the funnel process.

In our example here, we have a Two-Page Funnel: Landing Page that goes to a Thank You page. Additional pages that are required would just be sub-pages but aren't a part of the actual "funnel". What I mean by that is the potential customer doesn't have to go through those pages to move onto the next step in our process. These pages would be links at the bottom of the page in the footer section: Privacy Policy page and a Terms & Conditions page.

I know you may be wondering what does a Two-Page Funnel have to do with the One Step Funnel Program, don't the two cancel out the other? I mean, I thought it was "One Step"?

It still is, what I mean by "One Step Funnel" is that the potential customer or new lead, only has to do one thing. They have to complete "One Step" and that is to submit their contact information. When they complete that "One Step", they will receive your offer, begin receiving two-way text messages, voicemail drops, emails and a call from the staff to get them to schedule an appointment to use that offer. Just because we have a Two-Page Funnel, doesn't mean the potential customer has to do anything else other than complete that "One Step".

Here's an example of what an Opt-In Funnel will look like:

OPT-IN FUNNEL

LANDING PAGE **THANK YOU PAGE**

When we create your landing pages, we will always have people opt-in for your offer using a form. The form should be simple:

First Name

Last name

Phone Number

Email Address

The opt-in form will be set up with those fields in that order. You can swap first name and last name for full name, but we will need to have a phone number and email address with the name. You will have "experts" tell you to just get the first name and email address, since the less information you ask for, the more likely a person is to complete the form. Even though that is true, the difference in leads you gain will not be worth the information you give up.

After creating Ads for multiple different Industries, we have discovered that your conversion rates really only increase by about 10% by leaving out the last name and phone number field. If you ask me, I 'd rather have 90 leads with all that information, then a 100 leads with just a first name and email address.

Now that we know that the first step to Automation is having an Opt-In Funnel to send the Facebook Ad Traffic too. What happens when they fill out their contact information? That's where the second Automation Step comes into play, the Email Autoresponder.

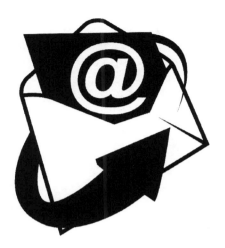

Automation Step 2: Email Autoresponder

"Ideas are easy. Implementation is hard." - Guy Kawasaki

For the most part, business owners know that they need to be collecting their patients' emails addresses and running email campaigns, but they just keep saying, "We'll get to it later."

For some Dental Practices, email marketing may seem old school. With the popularity of social media, and a number of other forms of messaging, the traditional email format feels relatively outdated. Even so, it continues to be one of the most used "modern" forms of communication. That's why almost every social media platform requires you to have an email address.

I believe that all businesses are aware of the importance of collecting email addresses for lead generation. Although email will ultimately only generate a small number of leads, it will build credibility with your potential patients. Yet besides the occasional email broadcast or current sales Ad, most businesses do not utilize the other part that email services offer.

I'm talking about the email autoresponder and in this Chapter I am going to talk about how we use it for our clients.

Before we begin, let's make sure we are on the same page on some terminology.

Email List: This is similar to a mailing list. It is a list of names and email addresses of a group of people. When someone fills out their contact information on an Opt-In Page, they will get added to a "list". It is likely, that you will have several different lists for your Dental Practice. We call these people on the list, "subscribers".

Email List Segmentation: This is an email marketing technique where we segment (or split) your subscriber list, based on any number of conditions. It is a technique used by businesses and marketers to send relevant communications to specific people in an email list.

Why Segment Your Email List?

The main idea of segmented email campaigns is to send relevant and targeted messages to specific people in the list. You can separate the list in a variety of conditions, such as buying history, age, geographic location, or previous email campaign interactions to develop relevant messages that will engage the subscriber. Most email providers allow you to "Tag" a subscriber and perform other "Actions" like add or remove them from a List.

The most effective campaigns start with qualified lists, so building a targeted email list should be your top priority. Even amazing email campaigns, with brilliant design, engaging copies, and unique value propositions can fail if your list isn't very good.

You should have three main priorities for building a quality list. In order, these are:

- **Quality:** You want real information from real people who check their email frequently.

- **Relevance:** These people should be genuinely interested in your services.

- **Volume:** If the first two priorities are squared away, you can start focusing on quantity.

Broadcast Message: A broadcast message is a single message that is sent to an entire list of people at the same time. It can be scheduled to go out on a specific date and time, but the schedule is the same for everyone.

Autoresponder: An autoresponder is different than a broadcast in that you can frame a sequence of emails that get sent out to the subscriber based on time. For instance, if someone decides to sign up to your list, they may get a series of emails sent over a period of time that will build a rapport between themselves and your Dental Practice and help them make a buying decision at a time when they would be most responsive.... when they first sign up.

Email Sequence: The "series" of emails are referred to as an "email sequence" and you can have as many different sequences that you want. You can have these be about anything you want that fits your business model. Maybe you have an informative sequence or a few of them explaining different services you offer and why they are needed.

Different Kinds of Email Sequences

Email sequences can advance people through a special journey of not knowing anything about your business, to becoming a customer and (possibly) an enthusiastic brand advocate. Email sequences can deepen the relationships you have with subscribers over time.

Why Email Marketing Is Still Effective

Email marketing has distinct advantages over other modern media.

1. It's direct, meaning that every person on your list receives an email the same way that they'd receive a piece of regular mail. It's much different than finding a piece of content in a newsfeed, even if it's personalized.

2. Email is necessary. You can go for a few days without checking social media or video chatting with your friends and family, but most people check their email several times a day.

3. It's highly customizable. You can create an email campaign on any subject and add any bells and whistles that you need to get the job done.

How We Use Email In Our Program

As far as scheduling appointments through email, we have found that it's virtually non-existent and doesn't happen that way. We use email to send that initial Discount Coupon to the new lead. We also use the Email Autoresponder as a way to build credibility with your new leads. In the Training Portal, we show you how to build out a series of emails that every new lead will receive regardless of how they Opted into your funnel.

Ok, so let's recap what just happened for just a quick second. We ran a Facebook Ad to our Opt-In Funnel (Automation Step 1). The person filled out their contact information (name, email and phone number) and clicked on the submit button. They were taken to the Thank You page to receive the special offer. In the background, upon clicking the submit button, that person was added to our email list and that triggered the

Email Autoresponder Sequence (Automation Step 2) to start sending out emails. The benefit of using an Email Autoresponder is that we can send emails automatically every time a new person signs up for information without having to rewrite them.

In the next chapter, we are going to talk about the "Conduit of Champions" and how this piece of our program links everything together.

www.OneStepFunnel.com

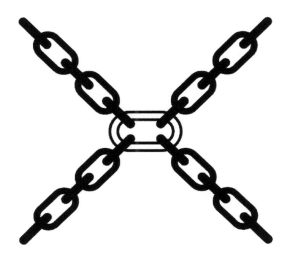

Automation Step 3: The Conduit of Champions

Automation Step 3 is probably the most important part in the whole process. It's what links everything together and makes it all work. There are a few different ways to go about this process, some are a lot easier than others and some will consume the happiness from your day. Yes, I have had this happen to me because of the way we used to do this step. That is, until we developed our own system.

In the old days, we had to download patient lists if that was even possible, manually add them to our Text Messaging software and we had to manually send a voicemail one at a time. There was no way to automate this process. So, having multiple touch points with a customer took a lot of time. Until now!

Now we can semi-automate the vast majority of the process. From when a customer Opts-In to our funnel and fills in their contact information, we can automatically send them an email. We can automatically add that person to a master contact list in a Google Spreadsheet, we can automatically send a series of Text Messages and voicemails over time too. We reply to the individual Text Messages, add the proper tags to each contact and book the appointments for our clients. All of that is setup and managed by us in the background while you are doing other things.

Think of the "Conduit of Champions" like a bridge connecting two things. It's like a big domino that once triggered, sets several different things in motion.

Let's start at the beginning, when someone fills out the contact information (Name, Email and Phone Number) on the Opt-In page of your funnel (Automation Step 1B), that "One Step" is the trigger that starts everything. As soon as they click the submit button, they will be sent to a Thank You page to get their special offer or discount coupon. Likewise, at the same time they are added to our email list and will start receiving your emails (Automation Step 2).

*** *Please note that each Automation Step is linked together so that its not too overwhelming to the person. We have all of the Automation Steps in a certain order so that they will receive them at specific intervals to not inundate that new lead.* ***

Simultaneously (Automation Step 3A), that contact is also added to a tab on a Google Spreadsheet that shows the date that person opted in, their name, email and phone number. This creates your "Master List" of potential customers. That is EXTREMELY important as most "Marketing Agencies" never give you this list, so this is an **Asset** you own! We will use this list for several things, but what it can also do is add them to a Direct Mail tab as well if you are doing these mailings.

We can also simultaneously in (Automation Step 3A), send a "Live Call Notification" to whomever you wanted to let them know you received a new lead and a reminder to call that new lead immediately.

Likewise, at the same time, in (Automation Step 3B), that contact information is sent to the Text Messaging Platform. I know this is the next Chapter, but you'll learn there that we can have a Text Messaging Sequence created, so that as soon as we add a new contact to that list, it would send a Text Message to that new lead at specific intervals. Also, this contact is added to the Ringless Voicemail Sequence as well, that's in a later Chapter.

Really, that's just the tip of the iceberg of what can be done with Automation Step 3, but I don't want to make things too complicated. I know this Chapter isn't very long, but I can't stress the importance of it enough, that this Automation Step is CRITICAL! It is the glue that holds everything together.

Automation Step 3 uses a specific service provider that includes our own built in Integration. We do that because for us to Automate all of the other tasks, we need this Automation Step to connect the Opt-In Funnel or Facebook Lead Ad to Our Platform.

In the next chapter we are going to talk about Two-Way Texting and the power of Text Message Marketing.

www.OneStepFunnel.com

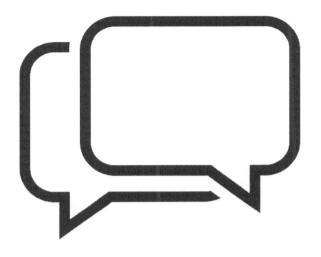

Automation Step 4: The Power of Texting

"You can't make anything viral, but you can make something good."
- Peter Shankman

I don't know about you, but when I get a phone call from a number I don't recognize, sometimes I'll answer it and other times I'll let it go to voicemail.

Have you ever received a Text Message from a phone number that you didn't recognize? Did you open it and read it? Chances are you did open and read it, and if you did then you would be like everyone else. You see, most people won't answer a phone call from a number they don't recognize right away, but almost everyone will read a Text Message from the same phone number. A Text feels safe and has a 98% read rate, meaning if you send a Text Message, it will get read.

How Does It Work

As soon as someone fills out the form on your landing page to grab your free offer, they got added to a Text Message Sequence (Automation Step 4) by the "Conduit of Champions" (Automation Step 3). That Text Message Sequence would immediately send a custom text to them within a minute or two of them completing the form? This is Automation Step 4 and this way, regardless of what's in the way of you being able to call them right now, our system sends a Text Message from you to them immediately! It will automatically address them by the name they gave in the form as well, making it feel more personal. I have an example below of what the Text Message may say if a man named John filled out the form:

"Hi John! Thanks for grabbing the $1,000 Off Dental Implants at ABC Dental. This is a limited time offer, so let's get you scheduled ASAP. Do mornings or afternoons work best for you?"

Once they respond, your team can respond back with the availability you have open and schedules the appointment.

On an ongoing basis, you will want to send out monthly Newsletter or Text Blast to your list, but only to new subscribers that way they are used to receiving a message from you once a month.

Two-Way Texting

On our platform, you have the ability to do Two-Way Texting. Many platforms use a short code, which is a 5 or 6 digit code that is the "phone number". Ever see a text from a "71441" or something similar to that? That's from a short code number and is a text message that looks kind of spammy.

On the system that we use, it uses a local phone number instead. That way it appears to be from a local phone number because it is. We can send automated text messages back in a sequence or send those one-time text blasts to your list. No matter how we use the platform, the customer can always respond back in an individual Two-Way Text conversation.

How We Use Two-Way Text Messaging

Our Platform will send the initial Text Automatically upon joining a Text Sequence when Automation Step 3B makes the connection. This connection happens almost instantly. In the Training Portal we will show you how to build out the Text Message Campaigns to engage with new leads and help nurture them to schedule an appointment. From there, we have set responses that your staff can use to help transition them from being a new lead to scheduling an appointment. A lot of this will run in the background, so your staff doesn't have to worry about responding to text messages individually.

In the next chapter, we will go over the second way we generate leads for our clients, by running "Reactivation Campaigns".

www.OneStepFunnel.com

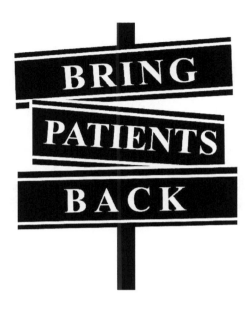

Reactivation Campaigns

There are no secrets to success. It is the result of preparation, hard work, and learning from failure." - Colin Powell

---

Have you ever seen an Ad from a Marketing Agency saying they can get you leads without any Ad spend? They may have used the words "Reactivation Campaign".

All this is, is taking your existing customer list, which is everybody you have ever done business with that you have a name and phone number for, and they use that list to import it into the Text Messaging Platform to send them a text message to "reactivate" them as a customer. The goal is to entice them to come back into your business. Maybe they haven't used your services in a few months, but by sending them a text message, you may bring them back in.

This is a very effective way to cultivate and re-energize past customers. You can have them take a poll, send them to a digital offer (Opt-In Funnel), ask them questions or remind them why they should come back to your practice.

I want to talk about the "Legality" of doing this. This is completely legal if you have created your database from customers either coming into your business, opting in on an online form, etc. Most people understand and expect occasional marketing messages sent to them when they provide this information to a business. That's also one reason we don't abuse this list and only send them one message per quarter, unless they engage with us through a Two-Way conversation. If you purchased a "list" from a third party, that list may not be used for Reactivation Campaigns because they haven't given you permission to reach out to them. That list should only be used to build custom audiences for your paid traffic campaigns.

How We Manage Reactivation Campaigns

The first thing we do is take a look at how many people are in your database. Most Dental Practices have a pretty decent database size, but it is dependent upon how long you have been in business. Typically, we see most Dental Practices have at least 2,000 people in their database.

What we have found is that cycling through your database once per quarter of a year works the best. So, depending on the size of your database that will determine how we cycle through that database and how much or how little we need to supplement lead generation with Facebook Ads.

What we typically do is get a goal dollar amount of new revenue per month, so we have a target to aim for. Let's say it's $30k per month. Then what we do is work the numbers backwards and start with the Reactivation Campaign and figure out what we think it can bring in. Then we supplement the rest with Facebook Ads like we did in the Marketing Budget chapter to reach that target goal revenue amount.

Behind The Scenes Of A Live Client Dashboard

One of my favorite parts of our platform is that it shows where everyone is in the process and the dollar amount at each stage. For example, the image below shows that we added 34 leads to this Dental Practice. We call them "Opportunities Added". To the right of that is "Pipeline Value", what that amount shows is the total dollar value of those leads. In this Pipeline, it's for the $2,000 Dental Implants Offer, so each lead has a value of $2,000. This shows that we brought in $68,000 worth of leads during this month.

Moving down the list, we have "Closed", that means that the patient came into the Dental Practice and had the service performed. This shows they had 19 Patients for $38,000 in Revenue! That's a pretty good month for most Dental Practices, but we see this quite often on our platform.

The next line is "Open", that is the number of leads that are either still in the nurturing stage or have an appointment that is scheduled. Those could still very well become "Closed" as well once they have an appointment.

Finally, the last line is "Lost", which means the patient had the appointment and decided not to have the procedure done. They would then go onto the nurturing step and continue to be re-engaged with over time.

Opportunities Added		Pipeline Value	
34		**$68,000.00**	
Closed	19	Closed	$38,000.00
Open	9	Open	$18,000.00
Lost	6	Lost	$12,000.00

Another great thing our Platform shows is the funnel view and the value of each stage in the process. These kind of metrics are important to see because it puts it into perspective for you and also shows you where people are at in your pipeline. It will also highlight where the "bottleneck" is and highlight those areas that need to be improved.

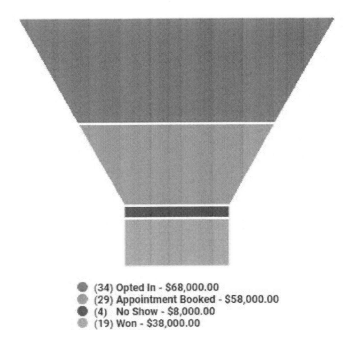

- (34) Opted In - $68,000.00
- (29) Appointment Booked - $58,000.00
- (4) No Show - $8,000.00
- (19) Won - $38,000.00

Similar to this chapter, the next chapter is about Ringless Voicemails or Voice Drops. These can and should be automated at first to have another way to reach out to new leads in a variety of ways.

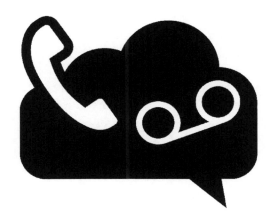

Automation Step 5: Ringless Voicemails

"Diligence is the mother of good luck." - Benjamin Franklin

Ringless voicemail also referred to as Voice Drops is a non-intrusive way to reach new leads and past customers with personalized, mass messages to get them calling your Dental Practice.

A few advantages of Ringless Voicemail:

- No interruptions to customers because there is no ring or just one ring.

- More likely to reach the targeted Prospect.

- Allows for professionally-produced, customized messages.

- Add the human touch to mass marketing messages.

Plus, it's also 100% FCC compliant!

Here's a fun fact, 90% of adults have a cell phone and 67% of those end up looking at their phone for messages, alerts or calls even when they don't notice their phone ringing or vibrating!

The rise in the use of cellphones has led to the decrease of traditional communication methods, which makes it more difficult for those still depending on those traditional methods to get in touch with people, to gather and share information.

This is where ringless voicemail comes into play (Automation Step 5). It is a cutting-edge technology designed to reach targeted audiences within minutes of sending. The clients we have on our system have had response rates as high as 12%.

Just imagine the ability to drop a voicemail message straight into the recipient's voicemail, without ever calling or ringing their phone line. There is never a charge for a call to the subscriber and the system is 100% legal. It is classified by the FCC as an "enhanced service" and is designed to be a non-intrusive form of communication.

Some systems allow the call to ring once, but then goes to the person's voicemail. Either way this is extremely useful because most people will listen to the first few seconds of a voicemail before they delete it, even from an 800 number. The system we use also uses the local phone number from the Text Messaging Platform, so this appears to be from a local number because it is. It is important to note that some phone carriers will not let these go thru, so expect about a 75% success rate when sending these out.

Ok, so let's recap how all of these Automation Steps work together to for the One Step Funnel Program. Originally, we ran a Facebook Ad to our Opt-In Funnel (Automation Step 1B). The person filled out their contact information (name, email and phone number) and clicked on the submit button. They were taken to the Thank You page to receive the special offer. In the background, upon clicking the submit button, that person was added to our email list and that triggered the Email Autoresponder (Automation Step 2) to start sending out emails. Simultaneously, our "Conduit of Champions" (Automation Step 3A) added that new contact to a Google Spreadsheet for our Master List of Contacts. Additionally, we had it (Automation Step 3A) send a notification to our sales rep or to whomever we have that is going to call this new lead immediately.

It (Automation Step 3B) also sent the contact information to our Two-Way Texting platform and added that new contact to a list there, which started the Text Sequence (Automation Step 4). At the same time, (Automation Step 3B) also added that contact to our Ringless Voicemail Sequence (Automation Step 5).

Not everything can be Automated through, in the next chapter we are going to talk about those non-automated tasks and your sales process.

www.OneStepFunnel.com

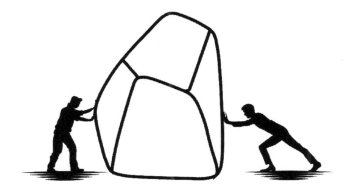

Non-Automated Tasks & Your Sales Process

"A goal without a plan is just a wish." - Antoine de Saint-Exuper

Although I just laid out a very successful system of Automation for you. A system that by its very nature will consistently nurture those new leads and help bring them back into your business. There is still one very important task that cannot be automated, the personal phone call.

The majority of Dental Practices don't do this at all. They pay a lot of money to generate leads and build systems to nurture that new lead, but seldom do they take that one extra step and call that new lead right when they are hot and ready to do business with you.

The Harvard Business Review found that 26.1 % of leads are followed-up with within 5 minutes, while the average response time for all leads is 42 hours. It's no secret that 35-50% of sales go to the business that responds first, so if a person is contacting you when they are ready to talk by submitting their contact information, why aren't we making every effort to speak with them immediately?

Dr. James Oldroyd published the Lead Response Management Study, which found that the odds of making a successful contact with a lead are 100 times greater when a contact attempt occurs within 5 minutes, compared to 30 minutes after the lead was submitted.

It's a rather terrifying statistic, but according to a study done for Harvard Business Review, 71% of qualified leads are never followed up with. What's more is, of the leads that are followed up on, they're only contacted an average of 1.3 times. Not only are we not focusing on these conversations, but we're quitting after just one call attempt?

As a marketing professional, my team and I work very hard to generate leads for our clients and it's to the company's benefit to ensure that these leads are being handled correctly. By creating a general process or "template" for your staff to follow, you are creating a more consistent and successful outcome. Below are a few ways to allow for better timing and consistency with your calls:

- **Create a series of scripted follow-up messages:** Keeping consistency among your team will allow you to determine which scripts work and why they work. I have my clients write up a short script of what to say to someone when they call that lead, that way no matter who calls on that lead the message is the same.

- **Get to know your leads:** Today, all different types of information can be tracked and measured; whether it be online, from a print ad, through unique phone numbers, or on social media pages. By knowing where your leads come from, you can determine what type of lead they are and react appropriately. Take the time to see where they came from and what they already may know about your company. Understand that some leads may know nothing about you (and this is likely their first visit to your site) and some will be returning leads with full knowledge of your products.

- **Adapt to the uniqueness of each lead:** Having different types of leads rolling in requires you to be well-versed in how to treat each one. Know that there will be differences between a form lead, a phone lead, or even someone who comes in from an advertisement. Each of these leads will require a different follow-up timeline with a script template customized to them.

- **Follow up in a timely manner:** Leads are like any other type of communication, in that the sooner you answer, the more likely you are to get a response. You wouldn't wait 3 days before following up on a personal phone message, and leads are going to be even more impatient. Set up criteria for each type and stage of a lead and generate a process for properly following up.

Fortunately, with Automation Step 3A, we can have one or multiple people notified that there is a new lead. That way you can have certain staff members calling this new lead on your behalf. It's important to have one person doing this at a time though so multiple calls from the same office aren't being made.

Click to Accept Call Feature and Call Recording

In our program, when a new lead fills out a form and submits their contact information during working hours, our platform will call your business to tell you that you have a new lead. The person who answers the phone can press a button and be placed on a brief hold while the platform calls the new lead to get them on the phone. This allows your staff the opportunity to schedule an appointment right away with that new lead and while they are most interested in your services.

During non-working hours, the person that gets notified will receive the contact information and will have a link to "Click to Call" that new lead. Depending on who or when they get notified, our clients can also use the mobile app to call the new lead and have the call recorded for quality assurance purposes. This is a great option to have to do spot checks on your staff to make sure they are following a script and speaking to your patients the way that you want them too.

So, When Do You Call and How Often?

I have my clients call the lead immediately when they get the notification. If the person answers the phone, then the staff member follows the script and tries to Schedule the Appointment in our Platform. If the person doesn't answer the phone, I don't have them leave a message and we call them back in an hour. If on the second call, they don't answer, I still don't have the staff leave a voicemail. Chances are the person will see two "missed calls" and will reach back out to you. If they do, then the staff member would try to schedule the appointment on our Platform.

On Day 2, if the person has not called us back, I have the client check our Platform to make sure the lead didn't book an appointment through our Automation Steps. If not, then we call them mid to late morning. If no answer, leave a voicemail. By this time, our regular Automation Steps are already taking over in the background as well.

On Day 3, repeat Day 2's activities. Make sure you are recording all activity for all days in a Google Spreadsheet.

But Doesn't This Response Time and Cadence Feel Creepy?

There certainly was a time when we thought this may be true. What would a lead think if they got a phone call immediately after submitting an online form? It would appear like we have absolutely nothing to do but sit by the phone and answer it!

But isn't that the type of service we're all searching for? If I've submitted a form on a website, it means I'm interested in more information. In this day and age where we all want information now and instant gratification is becoming an expectation, this would set you apart from your competitors. It's important that your call script be inviting and not pushy, this will add an element of success to the program.

Improving Your Sales Process

Since it's impossible for me to know what your sales process is compared to someone else's, I will say that successful businesses have a consistent process. What I mean by that is they have a plan on how they sell their services.

I strongly advise for you to have a sales script. If you don't have one, create one so that everyone is using the same script. This will make it easier for everyone to increase their sales. Sales scripts are often continuously refined or edited, that's okay.

A good script covers what questions to ask and when to ask them. If you are doing all the talking, then you are doing too much selling. A good sales strategy is to have the person sell themselves on your business, not you convincing them. You should also include your typical objections in your script as well. That way you can practice those responses, so they become second nature to you.

I can hear you saying to yourself that a "sales script in my Dental Practice wouldn't work". I beg to differ, because all the Dentists we work with have a script. One of our Dentists wrote a script on how to upsell a cleaning client to their teeth whitening service. In fact, all of his technicians use the same script when the patient appears to be a good fit. Once we added a script to his practice, they quadrupled the number of teeth whitening services that year.

Figure out what your sales process looks like and write up a script for each procedure. The next step is to rehearse that script with someone until you can deliver it without looking at the paper. That is what will make the most impact on your sales process than anything else. The goal is to continuously get better at sales. Your first draft of your sales script will not be very good. But, until you have delivered your sales script to over 20 people, at a minimum, don't make any changes. After 20 people, make minor changes, then restart the process and deliver the new sales script to 20 people.

Have You Ever Said This?

"I know how to sell. If I can get someone in front of me, I'll close 8 or 9 out of 10 times. I just need more people to know we exist."

Usually when someone says this (which is almost every time the conversation shifts to their sales ability), my next question is "where do most of your leads come from now?" Proudly, every one of them says "word-of-mouth" or "referrals". They say it proudly as they know it defines how good they are at what they do. Every single one of them say the same thing though!

Here's the thing, if all your leads come from referrals and you only close 9 out of 10, then you've got a sales problem. How did you lose that one person??? They came to you ready to buy!

Internet leads are a very different story and have a very different closing ratio.

"I'm not a pest. If they don't want to call me back after I call 2 or 3 times, I'm not going to beg them to come in."

At least 80% of all sales are made between the 5th and 12th contact or touch, yet more than 80% of sales people quit calling after the 3rd attempt.

You need to get resourceful. Are you texting? Are you emailing them? Are you inviting them in for your free offer? Are you calling them until they ask you to stop? It's all about "touch points", the more "touches" we can make the more likely it is for us to reach that person. My team doesn't stop until we get either a "yes" or a "no". If it's a "no", that means it's a "no, not right now" and that person goes onto a slow-paced nurturing program.

You will be surprised to find out that most people will thank you for continuously following up and not giving up on them.

"I need better leads."

No, you don't. You need more of them, and a better sales process. I hate when I hear people say, "I'd rather have less leads, but better quality, then more leads at a lower quality. Are you crazy? Get both!

Here's the way I look at it. If you and I each get 100 leads and closed 10% of them, we gained 10 sales. You can't stand that you didn't close 90 of them right off the bat. And because you've convinced yourself that you're incredible at sales, you point to the lead quality being poor.

If you're closing 10% of your internet leads, you're doing a great job! But if you chop that down to 20 leads so you can have people further down the funnel and find a way to close 10 of them, your ratio jumps to 50% and you feel great about yourself!

I, on the other hand, will spend more and get 200 leads and close 20, that's still only 10%. I've doubled your sales total and more than 10 X'd the amount of leads that now know who I am, what I do, and where I do it. This also gives me more people to follow up with, and overtime many of those will convert. You won't have that. And in 18 months, you and I aren't even in the same league anymore.

"I need better salespeople."

Sometimes this is the case. You must train your sales people every day. They must roleplay! Sales is hard, and they must be set up for success. Using a script and practicing this daily can take a horrible salesperson and turn them into an average salesperson. Likewise, it can take an average salesperson and turn them into a great salesperson.

"I'm a Dentist, we don't do "sales", we prescribe a solution to their problem."

Actually, you do "sales" all the time and you don't even know you are doing it. What makes your Dental Practice different than the one down the street from you? Why wouldn't a patient get a few "opinions" before doing a larger procedure? The answer is, how you sell them on your practice and what makes you the best solution to their problem. That is all part of the "sales process". Get better at that and I can guarantee you that you will have higher close ratios.

In the next chapter, we are going to talk about Automation Step 6: Getting Online Reviews! We will assume that through our Automation Steps and the phone calls the staff made to that new lead, that they came in for their appointment and that you were able to make the sale.

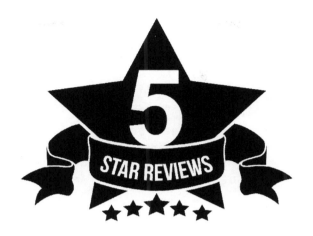

Automation Step 6: Get Online Reviews!

"Your most unhappy customers are your greatest source of learning."
- Bill Gates

Online Reviews may look like a straight-forward subject. However, most Dental Practices vastly underestimate the importance that online reviews have on their business.

In this day and age, it's never been easier for potential customers to discover what others think about your business.

This is both good and bad (depending upon what people are saying about you and what they see). People search online before they buy, and we realize that they put a lot of stock in what they find and read online. In fact, a recent Nielsen study shows that 74% of US Consumers choose to do business based on online feedback - even when it's feedback from complete strangers!

According to Nielsen's summary of their poll data, recommendations from personal acquaintances and opinions posted by customers online are "the most trusted forms of advertising".

Whether it is positive or negative in nature, most of the content about your business that is available online is not even being created by you anymore! Consumers are critics and publishers now. They all carry small "printing presses" in their pockets called cell phones!

Dental Practices have always depended on their reputation, but the stakes are even higher today, as a result of how easy it is for consumers to find information about local businesses before they buy.

We like to focus on Google Reviews in particular, and we suggest taking a practical approach to get them due to recent changes Google has made.

Google is often the first point of contact between a customer and a business. From finding businesses nearby, to looking up your telephone number, you customers will plug keywords into Google to help them find anything they want to know. And if they wish to discover how your practice compares to another, they will "Google it" to find out about other people's experiences.

Google Reviews are favored by the search engine and show up upon every relevant results, if your business wants to have a good presence on Google, best place to start is by getting more Google Reviews.

The importance of Google Reviews:

Getting reviews from your customers has always been a beneficial exercise for businesses, but today its importance is even greater.

There are three main benefits of getting customer reviews:

1. To acquire reviews, you can use in marketing your business.

2. To better understand your client's needs and how to serve them better.

3. To improve visibility of your business on Google.

The Power of a Few, Should Not Be Underestimated

The power of the customer review should not be ignored and its influence on other potential customers. You can tell me you are the very best Dentist in your area, and I might believe you. Having said that, if an impartial third-party tells me you are the best, I 'd be a lot more likely to believe it. In fact, one recent study found that 88% of consumers look for reviews before purchasing something, and yet another study indicated that 63% of consumers are very likely to make a purchase from a business that gets good customer reviews.

One fear reluctant business owners have in getting online reviews is the fear of receiving a negative review. However, receiving the odd negative review is not always a bad thing. Actively responding to bad reviews and trying to resolve the situation, illustrates to your new potential customers that you care about your clients.

A study actually found that bad reviews can increase conversion rates by up to 67% if handled appropriately.

So, Why Are Online Reviews So Important In A Local Marketing Strategy?

In Google's quest to provide the most relevant and useful results for local searches, they not only need to know what your business does but how your business is actually perceived. They accomplish this, in a big way, by seeing the number of reviews your business has and what your average customer rating is. Want proof? The Google Tour explaining the features of the new Google Maps states that the "highest rated" businesses near you will be returned when you search with local intent.

Google improved its map layout to show ratings and reviews a lot more prominently. The quality and quantity of reviews on Google is among the most important ranking factors for local businesses. If your search result listing shows a 4.5-star rating with 35 reviews and your competitor listings have less reviews, that's good social proof that your business is credible.

Even when reviews are not posted to your website, there are several websites like Yelp, Facebook, Google Maps and other social media sites where views will show up. To take full advantage of the fact that you need reviews and maintain as much control over them as you can, asking your customers to leave reviews about your business should be a top priority.

Impact on Search Results

Reviews have an added benefit in that search engines (such as Google) give extra attention to review sites. When a business listing, on Yelp, Google Maps and other review sites has reviews, the search engines will list them higher in the search results. Hence, the reputation of a business is highlighted by the search engine. Several elements combine to increase the search results of review sites. These include the overall rating, the number of reviews for the business, the number of recent reviews, consistent NAP (name, address, phone number), and the key words within the reviews.

Likewise, according to Google, the number of reviews and your overall review score affect a business's local ranking, which includes both positive and negative reviews. In fact, recent studies show that reviews round out the top seven factors in determining your ranking and can have as much as a 10% impact.

Acquiring 5-star Google & Facebook reviews can be a challenge, but with the One Step Funnel Program, we have ways to Semi-Automate this entire process and take your Reviews to a whole new level.

This completes the Automated System that we use for our clients and it works! In the next chapter, we put everything together to show what the One Step Funnel Program looks like. Check it out!

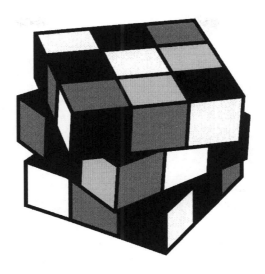

Putting It All Together

Congratulations!! You made it to the chapter that brings it all together into one well thought out system. To start this chapter off, I'm going to briefly recap how all six Automation Steps work together. Then, I'm going to show you piece by piece how all the Traffic Strategies, the Automation Steps and Online Reviews all fit together into the One Step Funnel Program.

If you recall, originally in our example, we ran a Facebook Ad (Automation Step 1A) to our Opt-In Funnel (Automation Step 1B). The person filled out their contact information (name, email and phone number) and clicked on the submit button. They were then taken to the Thank You page to receive the special offer.

In the background, upon clicking the submit button, that person was added to our email list and that triggered the Email Autoresponder Sequence (Automation Step 2) to start sending out emails.

Simultaneously, our "Conduit of Champions" (Automation Step 3A) added that new contact to a Google Sheet for our Master List of Contacts.

Additionally, we had (Automation Step 3A) send a notification to our sales rep or to whomever we have that is going to call this new lead immediately.

It (Automation Step 3B) also sent the contact information to our Two-Way Texting Platform and added that new contact to a list there, which started the Text Sequence (Automation Step 4).

At the same time, (Automation Step 3B) also added that contact to our Ringless Voicemail Sequence (Automation Step 5).

The Platform We Use

We utilize our own platform called the *"Patient Booking System"*. Our clients get access to this once we have the Automation Steps built out and customized to their Dental Practice. It's great for staff to be able to move patients into different stages of the pipeline and send the email or text message out asking for an Online Review after a procedure is completed.

Our clients also get access to the Mobile App, which they can download from the Apple Store or Google Play Store. This gives them 24 hour access to their marketing pipeline and the ability to respond to patient questions anytime.

PATIENT
BOOKING
SYSTEM

One Step Funnel Diagram

Now that we reviewed how all of these Automation steps fit together, let's go over piece by piece how all the Lead Generation Strategies, the Automation Steps and Online Reviews all fit together into the One Step Funnel Program. Here is a complete look at how everything fits together.

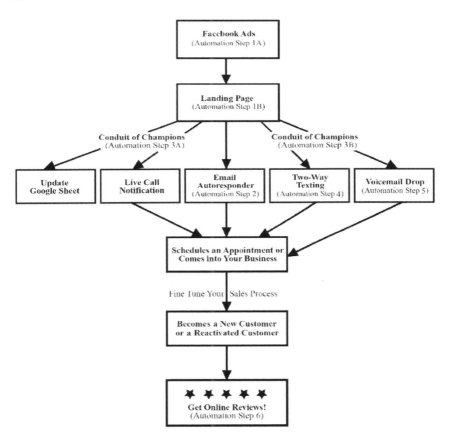

Automation Step 1A: Facebook Ads

In the image below, you will see a diagram showing you how a Facebook Lead Ad would be used in the One Step Funnel Program.

Once a person clicks on our Facebook Lead Ad, a window would popup allowing the person to click on the prepopulated information on the lead form. We could either give them the Discount offer coupon from there or have them redirected to the Thank You page we created.

From there, it's pretty standard for our Program, upon clicking the submit button, that person would be added to our email list and that would trigger the Email Autoresponder Sequence (Automation Step 2) to start sending out emails.

Simultaneously, our "Conduit of Champions" (Automation Step 3A) added that new contact to a Google Sheet for our Master List of Contacts. Additionally, we had (Automation Step 3A) send a notification to our sales rep or to whomever we have that is going to call this new lead immediately.

It (Automation Step 3B) also sent the contact information to our Two-Way Texting Platform and added that new contact to a list there, which started the Text Sequence (Automation Step 4).

At the same time, (Automation Step 3B) also added that contact to our Ringless Voicemail Sequence (Automation Step 5).

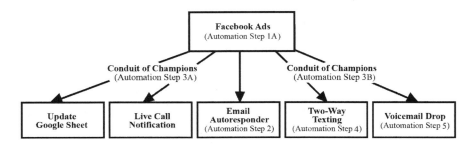

Automation Step 1B: The Opt-In Funnel

In the image below, you can see that we send our Facebook Ad traffic to the Landing Page. The Landing Page is the first page of our Opt-In Funnel and once a person takes action on this page by submitting their contact information (Name, Email and Phone Number), that "One Step" will trigger the start of all the other Automation Steps. The important thing here is to make sure your "Ad content" (Bait) matches the Landing Page content and vice versa, that way a person gets what they clicked on.

In the background, upon clicking the submit button, that person was added to our email list and that triggered the Email Autoresponder Sequence (Automation Step 2) to start sending out emails.

Simultaneously, our "Conduit of Champions" (Automation Step 3A) added that new contact to a Google Sheet for our Master List of Contacts and it sent a notification to our sales rep or to whomever we have that is going to call this new lead immediately.

It (Automation Step 3B) also sent the contact information to our Two-Way Texting Platform, which started the Text Sequence (Automation Step 4). At the same time, (Automation Step 3B) also added that contact to our Ringless Voicemail Sequence (Automation Step 5).

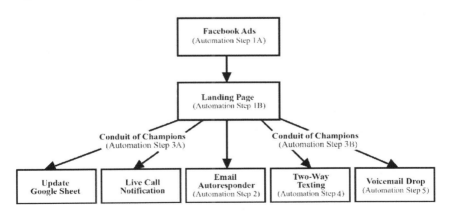

Reactivation Campaigns

In the image below, you can see how a "Reactivation Campaign" works. Basically, we take the existing customer list and spread it out over 12 weeks and initiate a Two-Way Text Sequence asking them in they would be interested in our special offer.

From there, we will nurture those that respond back to try to get them to schedule an appointment and show up to that appointment. Like with any Text Campaigns that we do, if someone asks us to stop sending messages to them or anything like that, they would be automatically unsubscribed from the list, so we don't message them again.

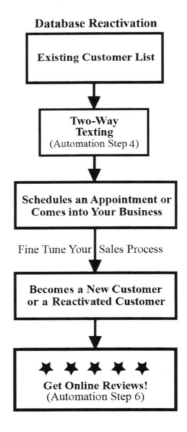

Database Reactivation

Existing Customer List

↓

Two-Way Texting
(Automation Step 4)

↓

Schedules an Appointment or Comes into Your Business

Fine Tune Your Sales Process

↓

Becomes a New Customer or a Reactivated Customer

↓

★ ★ ★ ★ ★
Get Online Reviews!
(Automation Step 6)

Email Autoresponder (Automation Step 2)

In the image below is how Automation Step 2, the Email Autoresponder works. Basically, when someone submits their contact information (Name, Email and Phone Number) and clicks the submit button on the Landing Page, that starts Automation Step 2.

By clicking the submit button, that persons contact information gets added to a list with the Email Service Provider. We also add a "Tag" to that new contact in the dashboard, that way we will know how they became a subscriber and we can market to that person again based on that "Tag".

When that new lead gets added to the Email List, that triggers an Email Sequence to start and that new lead will start receiving your emails automatically.

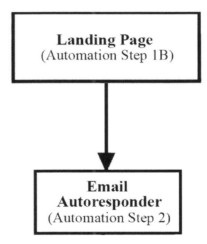

Conduit of Champions (Automation Step 3A)

The Conduit of Champions Automation Step 3 is broken into two parts. Automation Step 3A and 3B. Below is the first part, Automation Step 3A, which is updating a Google Sheet and a Live Call Notification.

Update the Google Sheet

As soon as someone clicks the submit button on the Landing Page, that triggers Automation Step 3A. The Conduit of Champions will update a row on a Google Sheet with that persons contact information. This is important to have for future Reactivation Campaigns and Facebook Audiences. Plus, its important to have an ongoing list of leads.

Live Call Notification

As soon as someone clicks the submit button on the Landing Page, that triggers Automation Step 3A. The Conduit of Champions will send a Live Call Notification to let someone know that you received a new lead and to call them right away. If this is setup through a Text Notification, then we can use the "Click to Call" feature, making this even more Automated. We have seen a tremendous improvement in Live Calls being made when we use the "Click to Call" feature. We advise them to be logged into the Platform to be able to schedule the appointment if they get a hold of that new lead.

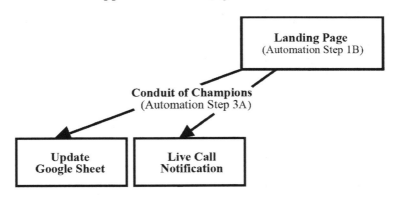

Conduit of Champions (Automation Step 3B)

The Conduit of Champions Automation Step 3 is broken into two parts. Automation Step 3A and 3B. Below is the second part of that Automation Step, which adds that new lead to the Two-Way Texting list and Voicemail Drop List on our Platform.

Two-Way Texting (Automation Step 4)

As soon as someone clicks the submit button on the Landing Page, that triggers Automation Step 3B. The Conduit of Champions will send that new contact information to the Two-Way Texting Platform and add that new lead to a Text Messaging List, which will start the Text Sequence.

Voicemail Drops (Automation Step 5)

As soon as someone clicks the submit button on the Landing Page, that triggers Automation Step 3B. The Conduit of Champions will send that new contact information to our Platform and add that new lead to a Voicemail Drop List, which will start the Voicemail Drop Sequence.

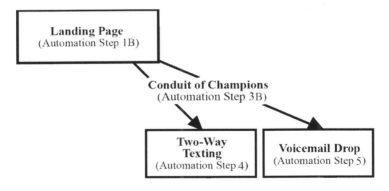

Now that you know how all the Automation Steps work together, let's see what the follow-up process will look like.

Automation Does The Follow-Up

In the image below, I want you to see how all of these Automation Steps work together to accomplish just one goal. That goal is to get that new lead to schedule an appointment with your Dental Practice and to show up to that appointment.

Please note, that your staff is responsible for making the Live Calls to the new lead. Our system will send a Live Call Notification, but its up to you and your staff to make the calls.

The Email Autoresponder, the Two-Way Texting and Voicemail Drops will all be automated and begin following their respective sequences.

My staff will respond to the Two-Way Text conversations on your behalf to try to schedule the appointment for you.

They say, "The Fortune is in the Follow-Up" and that's what really makes our system one of the best for Dental Practices.

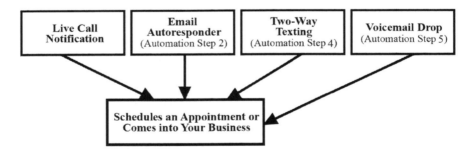

Becomes a New Customer

At this point in the process, the new lead has scheduled an appointment and has shown up to that appointment. Now its just time for you to sell your services. If they purchase your service, then you would move that person to the "Won" folder in the dashboard of our Platform. If they didn't show up or you didn't close them, then you would move them to the respective folder in our Platform so we could continue to nurture that lead accordingly.

Becomes a Reactivated Customer

Again, this is all about your sales process. These appointments should be easier to sell because they are previous patients or people that have done something with your business in the past. Its what we call a "Warm Market", meaning they already know, like and trust you. Like the above paragraph says, you would move them to the respective folder based on what happens at the appointment.

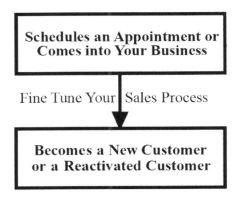

Get Online Reviews!

This is the one step in our program that may be partially "Automated", meaning it is automated, but your staff may have to manually trigger it to start depending on a few variables.

Since we have no way of knowing when a Patient actually completes a service or has the work performed, we don't want to send a Text Message to ask for a review until that work has been completed. Depending on the platform your Dental Practice uses, we can link our Platform into that so that way it will notify our platform to send a "Ask for a Review" text out automatically once the appointment is over.

So, if we can't go that route then for this step to work properly, we train the staff to ask the patient if they would be so kind to leave us a review. If the patient says "yes" or anything of that nature, then the staff member would simply fill out the online form and it would be automated from there.

We also continue to nurture that lead with our Reactivation Campaigns and follow up processes to bring them back in again in the future.

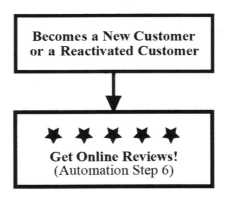

In Conclusion

I hope that you can appreciate the value that this system can bring to your Dental Practice. It is very complex, but that new potential patient only had to take One Step for our system to take over from there. It truly is a work of art when all the systems work in perfect harmony together. I am very proud of the way this system came together and is working for our clients.

Where To Get Help Setting This Up

You can get more information about the One Step Funnel Program at: **www.OneStepFunnel.com**

As a way to say Thank You, I wanted to give you something special to help you succeed even more and to show my commitment to your success. There is nothing more precious than time, so I would like to invite you to go to **www.OneStepFunnel.com** and Schedule a FREE Strategy Session with one of our Team Members.

If you are a good fit for the program, then we will figure out the best way for us to work together. No matter what you decide to do, take action!

In the next chapter we are going to go over some of those negative thoughts that are stopping you from taking action and how to overcome them.

www.OneStepFunnel.com

DON'T BE
THAT GUY
OR GAL

Don't Be That Guy or Gal

"The stars will never align, and the traffic lights of life will never all be green at the same time. The universe doesn't conspire against you, but it doesn't go out of its way to line up the pins either. Conditions are never perfect. 'Someday' is a disease that will take your dreams to the grave with you. Pro and con lists are just as bad. If it's important to you and you want to do it 'eventually,' just do it and correct course along the way." - Tim Ferriss

---

In this chapter I want to address the common phrases I hear all the time from Dental Practices that haven't yet figured out how to do their Marketing. So here we go...

"I can't afford to advertise right now."

If you can't afford to advertise right now, then your business is dead or dying. The only way to solve most business problems, is to have more sales (Revenue). Without sales, there are no "operational issues" or "staff problems" or anything really, because you have nothing to do. I'm sure there are ways to advertise, the problem is are you willing to cut out those expenses that are more "wants" than "needs"?

Typically, when we hear this response, it's usually from someone that was just scammed by a "Marketing Agency" that did very little but charged them an arm and a leg. I'm sorry you went down that path, you know better now, but you still need to advertise. People can't buy from you if they don't know who you are and what you offer.

"Can you just set this up for me? I can take it from there."

The short answer is No. We will set this up for you, but we manage everything for you in the background. We do this because what we find is that one of the first things that Dentists and staff like to do is start changing and tweaking the Text and the copy and they end up changing what was working to what doesn't work. We know what works and we handle the lead generation for you.

"I need to talk to my business partner or spouse about this first."

One of the first things we ask when we start talking to a potential client that is interviewing to be a part of our program is if everyone who is involved in the decision is on the call. If they say "No", the call is ended, and they would need to reschedule so that all of the decisionmakers are on the call at the same time.

If they say "Yes", we ask again with the clarification that at the end of the call, if they are a good fit for our Program, then we will extend a one-time offer to work together. If at that point they say they have to talk it over with a "business partner" or "wife", etc. then we may push back a little and dig deeper to find the reason they are saying that now. We do that because we asked twice if all the decisionmakers are on the call and they told us yes earlier in the call. There is either a different reason they have hesitation to starting to work together and we will dive into that or we may rescind our offer to work together and end the call.

We make it very clear at the beginning that the call is to figure out how we can help them grow their Dental Practice and see if our Program is a right fit for them or not. If they are a good fit for our Program, then we will extend a one-time offer to work together.

"This won't work for my Dental Practice."

This answer makes me laugh because they would need to tell that to all the other Dental Practices that use this system and tell them this doesn't work. Every business owner I have ever met, not even just Dentists, think that their business is somehow unique or different or special.

Here's the truth, its really not. Sure, you may offer something most people don't, but what we are talking about in this situation is getting quality leads for high end services for your Dental Practice. It's finding people that need your service and connecting the two of you. Nothing is unique or special in that, other than the location that we work with.

"Can I have exclusive rights to my city? Won't you just work with the Dental Practice down the street from me?"

We only work with one Dental Practice per area. That area does change depending on the size of the city, the population, etc. When we have a situation of an existing client and a new potential client, we look at the amount of leads we are currently getting for our existing client and whether or not we could support both to the full extent of our capabilities. If we can and they aren't right next to each other, then we may take on the second client. I will say that this hasn't happened yet and when it has come up before, we have turned down the potential client because they were too close to each other and it would make our existing client have less leads.

"Can't I just Google this information?"

Yes, you can, but it won't work the way it works for us. You could go out and find different platforms that do all the different Automation Steps and hopefully figure out how to tie them all together to work in perfect harmony. You may figure out how to run effective Facebook Campaigns and run Reactivation Campaigns. You could buy training courses that teach how to build Landing Pages and email campaigns.

Here's what we found in the past, that you will end up coming back to us because we have used all of those different platforms before ourselves. You know what we discovered? That there are always problems with something not connecting to the other. There are always missing pieces that for whatever reason stopped working and it took days to get through to support to get it fixed. This is why we ended up building out our own Platform to handle the bulk of what we need to do. We needed a solution to the ongoing problem of reliability.

I know the Two-Way Platform that's out there and how buggy it is. I also know of two lawsuits that are pending with that company due to Spam complaints and ruining a company's reputation and phone number. The FCC is not something to mess around with and when you cut corners to get a high volume of clients using your software, you put everyone at risk.

So, can you figure out how to make something "similar" work, maybe, but in the end, you will come back to us after it breaks.

"We need leads that have more money."

I've never seen so many people wearing "Air Pods" that costs around $160+ (thanks to Apple). No matter what age they are, people are spending $160+ on a set of earphones that does the same job the wired earphones do that come free with most devices. Think about it for just a minute and you will realize that the Air Pods don't solve any pain points that they've been dealing with. Most people also spend $500-$1,000 on a cell phone that does the same job as one 1/4 of the price if they were willing to settle.

Apple convince them they needed the Air Pods and new Phone. You did not.

You just have to remember who you're competing with. You're not competing with other local dentists. You're competing with everything else they want to use their paycheck for. Something tells me their fast food, coffee, movies, entertainment and restaurant costs will total more each month than your product or service would cost. That "broke" lead is getting sold by a cheeseburger better than you!

Long story short - get better at sales. What's the last sales book you read? How long ago? What about the one before that? Before that? How often do you practice sales? Do you role play with your team each day?

If you are reading regularly on sales, then great. You're feeding your mind new ideas and strategies that you can use. But practice with your team each day. Role playing is highly underrated, but the most successful Dental Practices do it every day.

"I have a website already, why do I need a Funnel."

In a previous chapter I talked about this briefly. The difference between a website and a funnel is that on a website it's not specifically geared to answer the reason the person got there in the first place. There are too many ways to lose a potential customer on your website. However, by using a landing page, which starts the funnel, you specifically address the reason that person came to your landing page. They have one action they can take on that page, either opt-in through your form or leave. That's it.

I like to use this analogy when talking to my clients. Imagine your website as a four-lane highway. There are several different off-ramps they could take, or they can continue going through your website until they hit a different off ramp. Typical off ramps on a website are the services page, blog page, contact us page, testimonials page, etc. These are great for informational purposes, but not to get a customer to take a specific action.

A funnel on the other hand, is designed for the person to take one specific action. This is like a one-way road. There is only one exit they can take and that exit appears when we want them to take it. Typical funnel looks like this: a landing page that has an opt-in form on it, which takes them to your offer page or thank you page. In this scenario, we created an Ad that when they clicked on it, they got sent to our landing page. On the landing page, they filled out a form, which got them on our list, and they were taken to the offer page or thank you page.

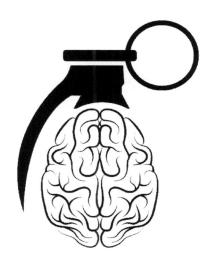

Knowledge is Power

"The value of an idea lies in the using of it." - Thomas Edison

If there's one thing I learned from all my mentors, it's this: education doesn't end because you're done with school. Especially when you start a new subject that school didn't teach you.

Which class did you take in school that really taught you the ins and outs of owning a business? How about managing and leading people, customer service, lead generation, business finance, marketing, advertising, sales, copywriting, operations, HR, taxes, laws, payroll, real estate, or any of the many subjects of business ownership and management?

If your school was anything like mine, you didn't learn any of that stuff. Without a doubt, you already got your hands in each of those areas listed above.

How's your practice doing? Is it ahead or behind of where you thought it'd be at the time of reading this book? The fact that you got to this chapter of a book that's designed to help you succeed, tells me you've got a fighting chance to reach your goals and destroy the competition that wants to take you down.

As hard as I worked on this book for you, I know it doesn't end there. You'll need to continue to educate yourself and learn, because you will always want to set new goals immediately after achieving the previous ones.

Final Thoughts

Thank you for picking up this book and I appreciate the time you took to read it till the end. I hope that you learned how an effective marketing system should be used to generate quality leads and nurture those leads to scheduling an appointment and showing up to that appointment.

Again, thank you for reading this book and if you would be so kind, I would really appreciate an honest review on Amazon for this book.

Also, be sure to go to **www.OneStepFunnel.com** and Schedule a FREE Strategy Session with one of our Team Members to find out how we can implement the One Step Funnel into your Dental Practice.

Thank you,

Adam Braithwaite

Marketing Terminology

Please note that not all of these terms are used in the book. I wanted to give you as many terms that I could so that you had a reference to go back to if you talk with another Marketing Person.

A/B Testing

This is the process of comparing two variations of a single variable to determine which performs best in order to help improve marketing efforts. This is often done in email marketing (with variations in the subject line or copy), calls-to-action (variations in colors or verbiage), and landing pages (variations in content).

Analytics

What I sometimes refer to as the "eyes" of inbound marketing, analytics is essentially the discovery and communication of meaningful patterns in data. When referred to in the context of marketing, it's looking at the data of one's initiatives (website visitor reports, social, PPC, etc.), analyzing the trends, and developing actionable insights to make better informed marketing decisions.

Call-to-Action (CTA)

A call-to-action is a text link, button, image, or some type of web link that encourages a website visitor to visit a landing page and become of lead. Some examples of CTAs are "Subscribe Now" or "Download the Whitepaper Today." These are important for marketers because they're the "bait" that entices a website visitor to eventually become a lead. So, you can imagine that it's important to convey a very enticing, valuable offer on a call-to-action to better foster visitor-to-lead conversions.

CAN-SPAM

CAN-SPAM stands for "Controlling the Assault of Non-Solicited Pornography and Marketing." It's a U.S. law passed in 2003 that establishes the rules for commercial email and commercial messages, it gives recipients the right to have a business stop emailing them, and outlines the penalties incurred for those who violate the law. For example, CAN-SPAM is the reason businesses are required to have an "unsubscribe" option at the bottom of every email.

Click Through Rate (CTR)

The percentage of your audience that advances (or clicks through) from one part of your website to the next step of your marketing campaign. As a mathematical equation, it's the total number of clicks that your page or CTA receives divided by the number of opportunities that people had to click (ex: number of pageviews, emails sent, and so on).

Content

In relation to inbound marketing, content is a piece of information that exists for the purpose of being digested (not literally), engaged with, and shared. Content typically comes in the form of a blog, video, social media post, photo, slideshow, or podcast, although there are plenty of over types out there. From website traffic to lead conversion to customer marketing, content plays an indispensable role in a successful inbound marketing strategy.

Conversion Rate

The percentage of people who completed a desired action on a single web page, such as filling out a form. Pages with high conversion rates are performing well, while pages with low conversion rates are performing poorly.

Cookie-Based Technology

Cookies are messages that web servers pass to your web browser when you visit a website. Your browser stores each message in a small file, called cookie.txt. When you request another page from the server, your browser sends the cookie back to the server. These files typically contain information about your visit to the web page, as well as any information you've volunteered, such as your name and interests.

Cookies are most commonly used to track website activity. When you visit some sites, the server gives you a cookie that acts as your identification card. Upon each return visit to that site, your browser passes that cookie back to the server. In this way, a web server can gather information about which web pages are used the most, and which pages are gathering the most repeat hits.

Cost-Per-Lead (CPL)

The amount it costs you to acquire a lead. This can range greatly depending on the offer, the targeting and the area.

Email

In its most basic sense, email stands for "Electronic Mail." It's a core component of marketing because it's a direct connection to a contact's inbox. However, with great power comes great responsibility, meaning it's important for marketers to not abuse the email relationship with a contact. It's far too easy for a contact to click "unsubscribe" after gaining their hard-earned trust in your communication. Don't blow it.

Engagement Rate

A popular social media metric used to describe the amount of interaction -- Likes, shares, comments -- a piece of content receives. Interactions like these tell you that your messages are resonating with your fans and followers.

JavaScript

JavaScript is what is called a Client-side Scripting Language. That means that it is a computer programming language that runs inside an Internet browser (a browser is also known as a Web client because it connects to a Web server to download pages).

Landing Page

A landing page is a website page containing a form that is used for lead generation. This page revolves around a marketing offer and serves to capture visitor information in exchange for the valuable offer. Landing pages are the gatekeepers of the conversion path and are what separates a website visitor from becoming a lead.

A smart marketer will create landing pages that appeal to different people at various stages of the buying process.

Lead

A person who has shown interest in your Dental Practice in some way, shape, or form. Perhaps they filled out a form, subscribed to a blog, or shared their contact information in exchange for a coupon.

Lead Nurturing

Sometimes referred to as "drip marketing," lead nurturing is the practice of developing a series of communications (emails, text messages, voicemail drops, social media messages, etc.) that seek to qualify a lead, keep them engaged, and gradually get them to schedule an appointment. Inbound marketing is all about delivering valuable content to the right audience. Lead nurturing helps foster this by providing contextually relevant information to a lead during different stages of the buying lifecycle.

Lifetime Value (LTV)

A prediction of the net profit attributed to the entire future relationship with a patient. To calculate LTV, follow these steps for a given time period:

1. Take the revenue the patient paid you in that time period.

2. Multiply that number by how long that person is a patient for.

For example, if a customer pays you $653 per year (ADA Average per year) and was a patient for 7 years (ADA Average is 7-10 years), then the patient's LTV is $4,571.

$653 per year x 7 years = $4,571

Marketing Automation

While there's some overlap with the term "lead nurturing," marketing automation is a bit different. Think of marketing automation as the platform with associated tools and analytics to develop a lead nurturing strategy. If you'll let me run with an "art" analogy, marketing automation is the paintbrush, watercolors, and blank canvas. Lead nurturing is the artist that makes it all come together. Like Bob Ross! You can't paint a happy little nurturing campaign without both.

Offer

Offers are the "bait" that we use to get someone to fill out a form on a landing page. Their primary purpose is to help generate leads for your Dental Practice.

Online Form

The place your page visitors will supply information in exchange for your offer. It's also how those visitors can convert into precious sales leads. As a best practice, only ask for information you need from your leads in order to effectively follow up with and/or qualify them.

Pixel (Facebook Pixel)

The Facebook Pixel is code that you place on your website. It collects data that helps you track conversions from Facebook ads, optimize ads, build targeted audiences for future ads, and remarket to people who have already taken some kind of action on your website.

Return on Investment (ROI)

A performance measure used to evaluate the efficiency and profitability of an investment. The formula for ROI is: (Gain from Investment minus Cost of Investment), all divided by (Cost of Investment). The result is expressed as a percentage or ratio. If ROI is negative, then that initiative is losing the Dental Practice money. The calculation can vary depending on what you input for gains and costs.

For example, let's say that you got $25,000 worth of business and it cost you $6,000 in marketing costs. That would be 316% ROI!

$25,000 in business - $6,000 marketing costs / $6,000 marketing costs

This book is NOT endorsed by Facebook in any way. FACEBOOK, Instagram and Messenger are trademarks of FACEBOOK, Inc.

This book is NOT endorsed by Google in any way. Google and YouTube are trademarks of Google, LLC.

Made in the USA
San Bernardino, CA
22 June 2019